YOUR CUSTOM IBS SOLUTION

HOW TO CREATE A PERSONALIZED GUT
HEALTH PROTOCOL AND DIGESTIVE WELLNESS
PLAN FOR IBS AND SIBO SO YOU CAN GET
YOUR LIFE BACK

AMANDA MALACHESKY

I'd like to dedicate this book to anyone suffering with a mystery health condition that doesn't neatly fit the conventional diagnosis model.

I see you, feel you, and have lived through the anxiety of not knowing what was wrong, and not knowing who could help me learn what the problem was, or how to fix it.

With some persistence and common sense, we can and will change how things are done, so patients everywhere can find a fast and helpful diagnosis.

TABLE OF CONTENTS

INTRODUCTION: WHY YOU NEED A NEW, CUSTOM APPROACH TO YOUR IBS

What if you had access to a strategy that showed you exactly what you needed to do to heal your Irritable Bowel Syndrome (IBS)? Would anything be different for you?

I know it may seem like a pipe dream.

As you've tried to find help for your gut symptoms, I'm sure you've scoured the internet looking for answers. To find solutions, you've spent thousands of dollars on specialized doctors, clinics, supplements, testing, and more. You've overhauled your diet (much to your family's chagrin) and tried to do everything the experts have told you, but many of you still aren't feeling well.

If this is you, I want you to know it's not your fault. But there is something important missing from your plan. It's not more supplements, testing, or tools, or a better doctor; it's guidance and strategy about *how* to use these tools you've learned about effectively. And though you may not know it yet, this is likely the critical missing piece that has prevented your success so far.

Your IBS Journey So Far (And Why You're Not Getting the Results You Want)

If you're here reading this, you or someone you love has been experiencing the challenging symptoms of Irritable Bowel Syndrome: bloating, abdominal pain, diarrhea, constipation, and sometimes nausea. It's upended your plans, kept you trapped at home, and maybe scared or worried you. Maybe it's gotten in the way of your marriage or partnership.

But the IBS issue that most frustrates me is how difficult and invasive it can be to get the diagnosis in the first place and how little help conventional medicine offers patients once they have a diagnosis.

If you're anything like the clients I've met over the last six years working with IBS patients, your gut journey has looked something like this:

Either slowly or all of a sudden, your gut started behaving strangely. More gas, bloating, or pain than you remember being normal is now your daily burden. Even worse, sometimes it's accompanied by embarrassing gas or too many trips to the bathroom that you don't want to explain to your boss or family.

In the beginning, you spent a lot of time researching on the internet, investing hours in blog posts, YouTube videos, webinars, and reels. After a while, the various influencers you met started to contradict each other. Who's right about which probiotics you should use, or which diet you should eat?

Next, you tried to put some of these options into practice. You spent a small fortune on supplements and tried using them, but noticed your symptoms got worse. Maybe you tried doing the low FODMAP or another diet, but all the food lists were different, and you didn't know how long you should continue. You asked yourself if this was really necessary.

Then, after weeks, months, or even years of struggling with

this, you finally decided to visit your doctor, looking for an answer about why this was happening and what you could do about it. Initially, your doctor likely recommended basic remedies, such as fiber, probiotics, or acid-blocking medication. You dutifully tried these options, but the fiber bloated you like a balloon, the probiotics were pricey and didn't do anything, and the acid-blocking medication made you feel crazy.

You went back to your primary care doctor, who finally referred you to a gastroenterologist (GI). The GI recommended surgical diagnostics like endoscopy and colonoscopy, and maybe blood and stool testing to rule out serious gut diagnoses. Sadly, despite extensive testing, your GI let you know that everything came out "normal," so you likely have "just" irritable bowel syndrome (IBS).

After this extensive workup, it can be demoralizing to be told, "You just have IBS." Once you have this diagnosis, you're likely to be told there's no cure, to be offered medications to control symptoms—and, if you're lucky, some information about diet changes that may improve your symptoms—but no help understanding your root causes.

And thus begins a long journey where IBS patients hope to find true relief so they can get on with their lives. But this help often doesn't arrive.

So if this standard approach to IBS doesn't help patients find relief, what does? Through my own personal IBS journey and my work supporting IBS clients, I believe I've uncovered a much more comprehensive and effective approach that helps IBS patients find their best long-term relief plan. It's not a one-size-fits-all prescription. Instead, it's a method designed to give you the tools you need to find real, lasting relief from your IBS symptoms. And the key to that comprehensive approach is *using the right strategy.*

My IBS Story

I learned about this strategy and method the hard way. When my IBS symptoms emerged, I was the mother of a young child, and my husband and I were building our own home on a remote 50-acre piece of raw land.

I don't know about you, but for me, there was nothing "just" about the symptoms I was experiencing when I was at my worst with IBS. On my bad days, I would have to cancel my plans, especially if it happened to be a day I was traveling somewhere. My pain would wake me up at night, and I could never predict what tomorrow would bring. Nausea, many bouts of diarrhea, fatigue, brain fog, and more became my frequent state of being. Pulling over on the side of the road for a gut emergency was not off the table. I began to limit my social outings because I knew I couldn't eat the food without paying for it the next day.

My time with IBS stretched out to years, and sadly, this isn't unusual, even when patients have a qualified gastroenterologist on their team. My access to help was limited, as were my finances, and I set out to do it myself.

I researched online to try and figure out what would help. The first diet I learned about was the keto diet: a low-carb, moderate-protein, and high-fat approach to food. The person promoting it claimed it helped all health problems improve. So I dove in, headfirst, and completely re-organized my family's diet and approach to food. This nutritionist gave me a supplement protocol for "healing my gut." It included around eight supplements, each costing about $15-$20, and I was supposed to use them for three months consistently.

The problem? The composition of the keto diet wasn't right for my gut or body, but I didn't know this. It made things worse, but slowly and over time, so I didn't see this forest for the trees.

I thought, "I'll just keep going a little longer because the benefits I'm supposed to get are surely just around the corner."

Those benefits never arrived, and I really damaged my gut health in the process. The supplements weren't necessarily right for me either, and I had no idea how to tell if they were actually helping. Meanwhile, I kept adding and trying new things that I also didn't fully understand.

After a few years of this, I decided to train myself to solve my problem. So, in 2016, I began studying Health Coaching, Functional Medicine, and Nutrition.

What happened next surprised me. I was sure I was on the brink of finding the solution I'd been looking for. I started applying what I was learning about functional medicine testing, nutrition, and supplements to my own case. But, despite having state-of-the-art tools and learning everything I could about lifestyle medicine, I actually continued to get worse!

So I started asking myself, "What am I missing to get better? If these tools aren't enough, what is?"

It wasn't until I studied Functional Nutrition with my mentor and award-winning Functional Nutritionist Andrea Nakayama of the Functional Nutrition Alliance that I figured it out: above all else, **true gut healing requires the right strategy and approach.**

The painful truth is that one-size-fits-all diets and cookie-cutter supplement plans are ineffective approaches for healing IBS. These plans overlook the most important question you can ask as you try and test new ways to improve your IBS: "Does this new [supplement, diet, or behavior] make my symptoms better or worse, and WHY?" The healing and success you desire is truly available to you by asking and answering this one simple question.

Your IBS Healing Road Ahead

You may be wondering if what I have to offer you in this book can really work for you. It's a fair question because I know it's highly likely you've been led to believe in many other things that have failed you.

My approach is different from just about any other gut health resource out there, and I believe that if you apply it properly, you can find your way to a healthy digestive system.

By studying the various options available for IBS patients, working on my own case, supporting my many IBS clients, and challenging the current medical knowledge of SIBO and IBS, I've created an alternative approach that I turned into an online coaching program. In the program, I help people suffering from IBS and SIBO find their personalized IBS relief plan that works. And now, I want to share that strategy with you in this book.

In the following pages, I'm going to share the strategy you need to not only find symptom relief, but also to know how to find an IBS relief plan that is tailored perfectly to your unique body.

In this book, I'm going to provide you with the critical information that can take you from IBS overwhelm, confusion, and frustration to an empowered relationship with your digestion and body. I won't just give you a list of diets or gut supplements but a strategy to decide which diets and supplements are right for you.

What I want to teach you here is *what* to do to improve your IBS and *how to use and sequence* the many IBS tools available. This next-level approach will allow you to make sense of the research you've done before and put it to work effectively as you find your root causes, create a custom IBS solution, and heal your gut.

What's important to me is that you're not only able to live without digestive symptoms but that you're able to pursue what's important to you. Maybe you'd like to travel, be a better parent to your child, or you'd like to be the husband, wife, or partner you've always envisioned. Maybe you have even bigger dreams, and your gut is getting in the way. Ultimately, the world is a better place when you're healthy and able to devote yourself to your passions.

Whether you're newly diagnosed with IBS or have been at this project for years, I want to offer you a message of hope. If you're willing to try this new way of thinking, I wholeheartedly believe you *can* find a personalized IBS solution. You can find a plan that either brings your symptoms into remission or, at the very least, teaches you what will best control and manage your symptoms in the long term.

No two people using this book will come to the exact same IBS solution. But you *will* find a unique combination of action steps that help *you* control *your* symptoms.

Let me help you find a peaceful belly and calm digestion, so you can live life fully and completely, without fear of accidents, embarrassment, or pain, and thrive how you were meant to. Let's dig in.

1

WHAT IS CAUSING YOUR IBS?

The million-dollar question you've likely been asking is, "What's causing my IBS?" I suspect you've wondered, researched, and worried as you tried to figure this out.

Conventional wisdom tells us there isn't a single, clear underlying cause for Irritable Bowel Syndrome, which is why it's considered a "syndrome." And though the symptoms can look similar among IBS patients, five patients with IBS may have completely different root causes. But I think you'll be relieved to know that while it's true that there isn't one single underlying cause for all IBS patients, there are often clear underlying *causes* that you can uncover and address in your specific case.

Let's explore what IBS is, and how to assess your most likely underlying causes.

Understanding IBS

Irritable bowel syndrome (IBS)—also known as a "functional gastrointestinal disorder (FGID)— is a digestive disorder that causes belly pain and discomfort and bowel changes. The word "syndrome" means that there is not a commonly accepted, known cause for these symptoms.

According to the Rome IV consensus (Rome Foundation, 2016), the defining symptoms of IBS are:

- **Abdominal pain** at least once a week for the last three months.
- **Changes in your bowel movements**, in either frequency, appearance, or consistency.

In America alone, between 25 and 45 million people meet the criteria for IBS (IBS facts and statistics, 2007). Women are the majority of IBS patients, but men also suffer from this disorder.

IBS should not be confused with Inflammatory Bowel Disease (IBD), which is caused by autoimmune damage to the digestive system. IBD is an umbrella term that includes Crohn's Disease and Ulcerative Colitis (UC). IBD patients may have IBS symptoms, but their IBS symptoms are usually coming from the clear cause of ulceration, inflammation, and autoimmunity in the digestive system.

There are three types of IBS:

Constipation-predominant (IBS-C)

You're pooping less than once per day. If and when you do have bowel movements, they can be difficult to pass, require straining, be hard and lumpy, or come out as small pellets.

Diarrhea-predominant (IBS-D)

You're pooping more than three times daily. Your bowel movements may be loose, fluffy, or liquid, have urgency, and be unpredictable.

Mixed IBS (IBS-M, sometimes called IBS-A for "Alternating")

You may have both constipation and diarrhea, either on the same day or on successive days. You may swing unpredictably between the two.

IBS can also include these core symptoms:

- Cramping
- Bloating
- Flatulence or gas

IBS is also associated with several non-digestive symptoms, including:

- Migraine headaches
- Chronic pelvic pain
- Reflux or heartburn
- Insomnia or sleep problems
- Fatigue
- Brain fog
- Respiratory symptoms
- Depression or anxiety
- Irritability
- Weight loss or weight gain

The Paradox of Getting an IBS Diagnosis

IBS is typically diagnosed when your doctor or gastroenterologist rules out all other possible digestive diseases.

To be fair to doctors, there are several serious gut conditions that need to be identified right away if they're affecting you. Most doctors are trying their best to make sure you don't have one of these severe diagnoses.

A few specific signs and symptoms would strongly suggest you need a more formal digestive system evaluation with your doctor or gastroenterologist. If you have any of the following symptoms, please do make an appointment to see your doctor and get evaluated right away.

- Blood in your stool.
- Mucus in your stool.
- Abdominal pain so severe you pass out.
- You're unable to keep food down.
- Feeling a lump or mass anywhere in your abdomen.
- You react to everything, even water.

These symptoms can align with colon cancer, bowel obstructions, Crohn's Disease, Ulcerative Colitis, gastroparesis, Mast Cell Activation Syndrome (MCAS), or many other possible diagnoses. These are all serious medical conditions that require prompt and proper treatment.

But now the IBS paradox: even in the absence of these signs and symptoms, if you present to your primary doctor or gastroenterologist with frequent digestive symptoms, they're likely to order the following tests to rule out these severe digestive diseases.

- GI studies, including endoscopy (stomach scope) and colonoscopy (colon scope).
- Blood labs to screen for celiac disease.
- Single marker stool tests, like calprotectin.
- Stool tests to screen for parasites, such as *Giardia*, or bacterial infections, like *C. difficile*.

Only if all these tests are negative does your doctor typically diagnose you with IBS. This simply means that despite your multi-thousand dollar workup, you have persistent digestive symptoms that specific gut diseases can't explain.

The challenge with this is that you still don't know what's wrong with your digestion or how to fix it. Just this morning, I met with an IBS patient with painful bloating, loose stool, and burping who had been to multiple gastroenterologists, but none of them had anything useful to offer.

This diagnosis model mostly tells you what you *don't* have. And while this can be a relief, many IBS patients are frustrated by their debilitating digestive symptoms and the battery of invasive tests, only to be told everything is normal. Research also appears to agree. For example, a 2021 study suggests that endoscopy and colonoscopy procedures don't find much of value for IBS patients (Staller et. al., 2021).

Through my work with IBS patients and my study of the syndrome, I know that there *are* causes that can be addressed. Ultimately, this is what you really need to know, regardless of the official diagnosis or label. So let's discuss what those IBS causes are likely to be.

A Short List of IBS Causes

Now that you have a formal (or suspected) diagnosis of IBS, the natural next question is, "Why is it happening?" Though the root causes of IBS won't be the same for every IBS patient, there is a short list of things that can cause IBS, and you *can* figure out which ones are affecting *you*.

The single, most common underlying cause of IBS is a condition called **SIBO**, an acronym for **Small Intestinal Bacterial Overgrowth.**

Dr. Mark Pimentel and his team's recent research at the MAST Program at Cedars-Sinai Medical Center in Los Angeles suggests that approximately 60% of IBS cases are caused by SIBO (Takakura & Pimentel, 2020).

The remaining common underlying causes of IBS symptoms include a relatively short list of problems. They include:

- **Non-SIBO bacterial dysbiosis or infections** (imbalance or overgrowth of bacteria)
- *H. pylori* bacterial infection
- **Intestinal parasites,** including amoebas or worms
- **Candida** or other yeast overgrowth
- **Food intolerances**
- **An overactive nervous system**
- **Poor function of your digestive organs,** including the stomach, pancreas, gallbladder, and intestines
- **Structural issues** (scar tissue and obstruction)
- **Endometriosis** and the adhesions and scar tissue it causes
- **Mold illness** (relatively rare, but possible)
- **Medication side effects,** especially from opioids

I'll detail these possible root causes and how to assess which ones are yours later in Chapter 6.

It's important to remember that you may have more than one IBS root cause. In fact, it's more common than not to have multiple, overlapping root causes. They're often interrelated. In my case, parasites, SIBO, endometriosis, AND food intolerances were all part of my root causes, and I had to address all of them to get well. My client Mike had oxalate sensitivity, yeast overgrowth, and Lyme co-infections. The point is to avoid thinking you're working to find the ONE single root cause because this may not be a reality.

In addition, some GI diseases can cause IBS-like symptoms. These are conditions that your doctor typically rules out with the previously mentioned conventional diagnosis path, but not always. If you haven't met with a doctor yet, or you think your doctor may have overlooked something, here is a short list of conditions that should be on your radar:

- Inflammatory bowel disease (IBD)
- Celiac disease (an autoimmune attack on the small intestine tissues)
- Exocrine Pancreatic Insufficiency (EPI)
- Autoimmune diseases, including Hashimoto's thyroiditis and Type 1 diabetes
- Diverticulitis/diverticulosis
- Steatorrhea (fatty stool)

The challenge is, which underlying cause (or causes) is *your* problem? This is the million-dollar question that I hope to help you answer with this book.

How to Figure Out *Your* IBS Root Causes

It's great that you have this short list of possible IBS causes, but this still doesn't tell you what's responsible for *your* bloating or diarrhea. Rather than trying to define IBS by what it isn't, like most doctors do, I've developed a systematic method to help my clients answer this question. If you don't have any clear warning or danger signs (see above), I propose an alternative approach to evaluating what's happening in your gut.

Teasing out your underlying IBS cause(s) from this list requires a structured investigation process. Your personal IBS causes could be any combination of underlying infections, food intolerances, nutrient deficiencies, stress reactions, or other causes.

When I don't know how to answer a question, I like to get methodical about building an answer from the ground up. And because of the complexity of IBS, it's key to get organized in your approach to make sense of it all.

Here is a 10,000-foot view of the method I developed for figuring out your IBS root causes. I call it "The Calm Digestion Method," and it's how I help my clients find their custom IBS relief plan.

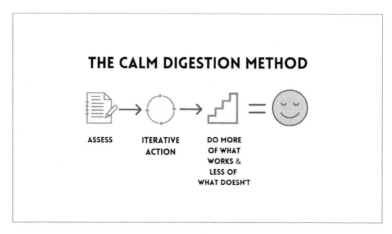

THE CALM DIGESTION METHOD

ASSESS   ITERATIVE   DO MORE
         ACTION   OF WHAT
                     WORKS &
                     LESS OF
                     WHAT DOESN'T

Figure 1: The Calm Digestion Method

The Calm Digestion Method

The Calm Digestion Method includes three main steps to help you figure out what's causing your IBS symptoms and what you can do to feel better. Here's a brief overview of each phase:

STEP 1: ASSESS (HEALTH HISTORY AND TESTING)

If you want to create an elegant solution to a complex problem, you must first understand what you have to work with. Your first step is to take stock of what you already know and use that information to make educated guesses about how your symptoms are being caused.

Many IBS patients I meet with are desperate for relief and want to dive right into *doing* something. In my first meeting with them, they'll say, "Please, what supplements should I start with to stop my constipation?"

I always answer that I don't know yet because we haven't yet done our homework to understand what problem they need to address.

It's also common for my incoming clients to be overwhelmed with what they don't know because the possible options seem almost infinite. I'd like to reframe this for you. The truth is that a few specific pieces of *what you already know* most often contain the clues you need to start getting better.

Whether you're just newly diagnosed with IBS or you've been suffering for years, there are four key questions to ask in your assessment that can help you get to the bottom of your IBS causes quickly:

- What was happening when you first got sick?
- What makes your symptoms better or worse?
- What did any recent test results show?

- What mechanism (more on this in a bit) might explain HOW these symptoms are being caused?

The answers to these questions help you create a short list of your most likely IBS symptom causes. Later in this chapter, I'll explain how to pull this information out of your medical history and how to use it to figure out why your IBS symptoms are likely happening.

Step 2: Complete "Iterative Action" Experiments

Iterative action simply means doing experiments to learn something and choosing your next steps based on what you've learned. I'm going to explain my signature Iterative Action Method in detail in Chapter 2.

You created a short list of the likely and suspected causes of your IBS symptoms in your assessment. However, we still don't know which of these possible root causes and symptom mechanisms are truly *your* symptom causes. So now you will trial and test potential therapies the right way to see whether your suspicions are correct.

This is where most people with IBS are taking action already. They learn about a supplement they haven't tried, decide to order it, and take it. Or they hear about a special diet that is supposed to help gut challenges, and dive in headfirst to try it out.

But they've usually skipped the assessment step, and aren't trialing these things correctly with the right questions in mind. They choose random actions without understanding why they're testing them or what they hope to address.

Done correctly, the results of your Iterative Action Experiments directly show you what your specific IBS causes are.

. . .

Step 3: Do More of What Works and Less of What Doesn't

After you've confirmed your specific IBS causes using Iterative Action Experiments, you then use what you learned to create a long-term management or maintenance plan by continuing to do more of what works and less of what doesn't.

For example, if you find that probiotics improve your bloating and constipation, then you keep using them. If you find that onions and garlic make your bloating flare up, then you avoid adding them to your meals. It really is this simple.

By creating a plan based on what you actually observe in your body, you create a custom IBS solution, designed just for you.

So let me start by teaching you how to assess your case correctly, so you can create that short list of your most likely IBS root causes.

Getting Started With Your IBS Root-Cause Investigation: Assessment

Though it's tempting to get started *doing* things right away to address your IBS, it's crucial to first assess your history and testing. Completing an assessment of your case correctly gives you the plan you need to begin testing therapies so you can find the right remedies for you.

As you read through this section, grab a piece of paper and pen or pencil, and jot down some notes. When you finish this chapter, you'll have a list of your possible IBS root causes.

What Was Happening When You First Got Sick?

The first question to ask yourself is, "What was happening around the time I got sick?"

I call these clues your original **trigger event**(s), which is simply anything that started your symptoms. They often help illuminate the original cause of your IBS symptoms.

Many of my clients report that their IBS started with a series of overwhelming events, like a divorce, a death in their family, or a period of financial strain. Another very common trigger event is a case of food poisoning. Lots of my clients tell me they were never the same after visiting a foreign country where they had a case of food poisoning or traveler's diarrhea.

Other common IBS trigger events include:

- **Hormone shifts** from pregnancy, birthing, lactation, or menopause.
- **Medication changes**, especially with opioids.
- **Major life changes**, such as starting a new job, getting married or divorced, a parent or in-law moving in with you, moving, a death in the family, welcoming a new child, a period of financial stress, or an illness, like influenza, COVID, or mononucleosis.
- **A diet change.** (Surprisingly, sometimes people develop IBS after trying a new diet that they thought was healthier. My client, Mary, had this exact situation when she tried to eat a "healthier" diet that was rich in fruits and veggies to prevent cancer, but wasn't tolerating the increase in dietary fiber. A simple return to less fiber and reducing FODMAPs helped a lot.)
- **Frequent antibiotic use.**

Note what you consider to be your top three or four initial trigger events on a short list.

Once you have this short list of initial symptom triggers, set the list aside. You'll need it again in a few minutes.

What You Already Know About What Changes Your Symptoms

Though you may feel confused about many aspects of your situation, I'll bet you're clear about a few details.

First, make a list of things you've noticed improve your symptoms. These could be foods, supplements, medications, or behaviors. For example, you might know that getting enough sleep, going on vacation, and using over-the-counter laxatives improve your symptoms.

Next, list the things you know make your symptoms worse. Again, these could be anything from food to medications or behaviors. For example, maybe you know that popcorn is horrible for you, the medication Linzess gives you diarrhea, probiotics make you feel worse, and your symptoms flare up whenever your stress gets worse.

You can also list things you've tried that didn't make any difference at all because you already know you can ignore these.

Jot these notes down and put them aside.

Testing

In the hands of a competent health practitioner, IBS lab testing can be a very valuable assessment. In addition to the standard testing your regular doctor or gastroenterologist may have ordered, there are three super useful tests for IBS patients. In an ideal world, these tests would be offered to likely IBS patients first, rather than subjecting them to invasive, expensive testing.

IBSSMART TEST: A SHORTCUT TO CONFIRMING IBS-D

What if you had a simple blood test that could confirm whether or not IBS is causing your diarrhea? The **IBSSmart blood test** is just that. Developed by Dr. Mark Pimentel's team at the MAST program at Cedars-Sinai, the test checks for two blood markers that can confirm an IBS-D diagnosis. (Unfortunately, this test doesn't help with IBS-C.)

A previous case of bacterial food poisoning causes a significant number of IBS diagnoses. The bacteria releases a toxin, called Cytolethal distending toxin B (CdtB). Exposure to this toxin can damage the nerves that regulate your small-intestinal motility. This toxin can also lead your body to develop anti-vinculin antibodies, which attack the nerves in the small intestine. The combination of this toxin and antibody can lead to the development of SIBO (Small Intestinal Bacterial Overgrowth) by reducing small intestinal nerve function and the natural cleaning waves in the small intestine.

The IBSSmart test checks for the CdtB toxin and anti-vinculin antibodies. If the test comes out positive, there is a 98% chance you have IBS-D and not a more serious digestive condition. If the test is negative, you may still have a different type of IBS, but this tells you that the cause isn't the bacterial toxin or anti-vinculin antibodies. The test has a 98% specificity and sensitivity for IBS-D, meaning that if it's positive, this is clearly the problem for you.

If you have IBS-D, it may be worth asking for this test to confirm or rule out IBS. See the Resources Section for information about accessing the IBSSmart test.

SIBO BREATH TEST

Recent research suggests SIBO (Small Intestinal Bacterial Overgrowth) causes approximately 60% of IBS cases. So if

SIBO is the single most common underlying cause of IBS, doesn't it make sense to test for SIBO early in your diagnosis process? Sadly, many IBS patients and their doctors are unaware of SIBO and the SIBO test.

The SIBO breath test is a simple, non-invasive, at-home or in-lab test to look for hydrogen, methane, and hydrogen sulfide gas produced by overgrown bacteria in your small intestine.

During the test, you drink a challenge solution, either lactulose or glucose. Then, you collect breath samples over two or three hours every 15 or 20 minutes, depending on the test. Only bacteria release hydrogen, methane, or hydrogen sulfide gas, so if these gasses turn up on your test in the first 90 minutes, this tells you that you have an overgrowth of bacteria in your small intestine.

Some critics of SIBO testing suggest that the test isn't accurate and shouldn't be used. And while it's true that the sensitivity and specificity data, which determine how accurate a lab test is, is not ideal, the test is still quite useful in the hands of a skilled practitioner. It's certainly less invasive and expensive than the "gold standard" test, where a fluid sample is taken from the small intestine while you're under anesthesia during an endoscopy procedure. In addition, Dr. Pimentel's recent research suggests that breath test results correlate closely with a small intestinal aspirate. This strongly suggests the breath test is an adequate stand-in to give you clinically useful information in a much less invasive way.

I recommend using the TrioSmart SIBO test, as it tests for all three SIBO gasses. You can contact the company directly if you don't have a doctor willing to order the test for you. If their screening determines you could benefit from the test, they will allow you to order one yourself.

The FoodMarble AIRE 2 home device also allows you to screen for gasses released by the SIBO bacteria and is about the same price as a single SIBO test kit but is reusable. At the time of this writing, the AIRE 2 device doesn't give hydrogen sulfide readings, but the sensor is already included in the device and should be able to take readings soon.

See the resources at the end of the book for how to access this testing.

GI MAP Stool Test

Many conventional doctors will commonly run a culture-based ova and parasite stool test if their patients are presenting with diarrhea. But these tests often miss other potential causes of IBS symptoms and very often miss subclinical gut infections.

DNA-PCR-based stool testing that looks for a wide range of possible gut irritants is helpful to see what else may be affecting your digestive symptoms.

The GI MAP Stool test is a home-collection stool kit offered by Diagnostic Solutions Laboratory. The lab uses DNA-PCR technology to screen your stool for over 70 microorganisms that may be affecting your gut symptoms. The test includes screening for common pathogens, like *C. difficile* and *Giardia*, yeasts like *Candida*, parasites, viruses, and bacteria that may cause symptoms. It also contains a panel of digestive markers often used by gastroenterologists to further refine their diagnoses of gut disorders, such as elastase-1 and calprotectin.

I find the GI MAP stool test extremely valuable in practice. It can help you not only rule out some more serious possible causes of your IBS symptoms, but it also often catches infections that other testing has missed. I commonly see this with *H. pylori* infection, the stomach-dwelling bacteria that can cause ulcers, gastritis, and heartburn.

Because these tests rely on DNA technology, they can find tiny quantities of the organisms they're looking for. Even better, they report their specific quantities. This way, even if the amount is below the "flag limit," we still know it's there.

Paired with the IBSSmart and SIBO test, the GI MAP rounds out the picture of possible underlying causes of your IBS symptoms. And because it includes stool markers that can help show non-IBS root causes without invasive procedures, I feel it's a valuable collection of screening to help you understand what's happening in your gut.

You're required to have a clinician order a GI MAP test. Diagnostic Solutions Laboratory can help you find a clinician near you who can order the test.

See the resources section for information on how to access functional stool testing.

If anything important turns up on your GI testing, jot those down on your notes along with your initial triggers, and things that make your symptoms better or worse.

Create a Hypothesis About How Your Symptoms Happen

At the most basic level, the critical question you want to ask as you test and trial things to help your IBS is, "*How* or why are your symptoms happening? What drives them? What makes them better, and what makes them worse?" I call this your **symptom mechanism.**

So next, using the lists you've just made, you're going to consider what physiological **mechanism** might explain your trigger events and the things that make your symptoms better or worse.

A **symptom mechanism** is simply the physiological reason your symptoms might be happening. You could also call your symptom mechanism your "**root cause**" or your "**underlying cause.**" Look at the items on the lists you just made and hypothesize about why you think those things are happening.

If you always bring your inquiries back to this focus, you will make progress with your IBS.

For example, if you know you feel better while on vacation, this might mean that stress is a mechanism of your symptoms, or that you're reacting to something in your home. If you feel worse from probiotics, this might mean you have SIBO, a histamine intolerance, or that you react to prebiotics (which are often in probiotic supplements). For an illness, immune changes or inflammation may be to blame. With medication changes, perhaps the medication's mechanism of action affects gut motility. Do some thinking on this subject, and ask your doctor or other trusted guide questions about what they think might have contributed to this shift in your gut health from your trigger. Here is a partial list of mechanisms of common trigger events and mediators:

Triggers	Possible Mechanisms
Menstruation, Pregnancy, Birth, Lactation, Menopause	• Hormones • Thyroid • Endometriosis
Medication changes	• Effects on motility • Effects on serotonin • Other medication mechanisms
Major life changes, Stress, Trauma	• Nervous system dysregulation
Illness	• Immune dysregulation • Gut microbiome change
Food poisoning/Traveler's diarrhea	• Motility damage • Gut microbiome change • Infections
Diet change	• Gut microbiome change • Difficulty digesting a component of the new diet (for example, fats or fermentable fiber) • Sensitivity to new ingredients
Frequent antibiotic use	• Gut microbiome change • Fungal overgrowth
Injury/Surgery	• Adhesions • Medication changes • Stress/trauma

Table 1: Common IBS triggers, and some of their possible mechanisms.

Mediators	Possible Mechanisms
Gluten	• FODMAP Sensitivity • Celiac disease • Allergy
Dairy	• FODMAP Sensitivity (Lactose Intolerance) • Casein (Dairy protein sensitivity) • Allergy
Kale and Nuts make things worse	• FODMAP Sensitivity • Oxalate Sensitivity
Monthly periods make symptoms worse	• Cravings cause you to make poorer than usual food choices • Hormone imbalance • Endometriosis
Going on vacation improves symptoms	• Stress • Mold in home or workplace
Raspberries, Chocolate, and Citrus make symptoms worse	• Histamine • High acid
Eating animal protein makes symptoms worse	• Low digestive enzymes (protease) • Low stomach acid • Slow motility

Table 2: Common IBS mediators and some of their likely mechanisms.

YOUR PARTICULAR LIST MIGHT LOOK SOMETHING LIKE THIS:

Initial Trigger: • Food poisoning in Nepal • Perimenopause • High stress	Possible mechanisms: • Parasites, motility damage (SIBO) • Hormones • Nervous system
Things that make symptoms better: • Sleep • Relaxation • Gluten free diet, dairy free diet	Possible mechanisms: • Nervous system • Nervous system • FODMAP sensitivity, lactose intolerance
Things that make things worse: • STRESS • Monthly periods • Gluten, dairy, sugar	Possible mechanisms: • Nervous system • Hormones • FODMAP sensitivity, lactose intolerance

Table 3: Summary of triggers, mediators, and their possible mechanisms.

Believe it or not, this list is precious gold on your quest to find gut relief. It shows you the most likely reasons your symptoms are happening and gives you a tidy list of hypotheses to begin testing. To start, you simply decide to take action to test one of these theories. That's a lot easier than swimming in an ocean of possibilities, isn't it?

Your possible IBS mechanisms are likely to fall broadly into a short list of categories:

- Stress and its effects
- Food intolerances or allergies
- Deficiencies in your normal digestive function (like poor gallbladder function or low stomach acid, for example)
- Underlying infections or dysbiosis (the testing I mentioned can help confirm)
- Structural abnormalities, like adhesions or restrictions.
- Medication actions

The point of this exercise is to narrow the field and provide you with a clear direction of action. Take some time to create your own unique list of triggers and mediators, and brainstorm about their possible underlying mechanisms. Once you have that list, it's finally time to start doing something about it.

In the next chapter, I'll help you understand how to use targeted Iterative Action Experiments to test your theories to determine which of these suspected symptom mechanisms are yours. First, I'll share the strategy you need to correctly experiment with stress relief, diet, supplements, and infection treatments so you can get the quality answers you crave. Next, I'll share the options that are most likely to help you.

Because there is no single root cause for all cases of IBS, your unique journey through this material will be particular to you. The pieces that are relevant for you may not be helpful for the next reader. I hope you can understand at this point that a unique combination of experiments will help you discover and confirm what's causing your IBS and what to do about it. If done correctly, you should be left with a relatively simple list of what's causing your symptoms, so you can take action to correct them. This is where we will be venturing throughout the rest of this book.

2

REAL-WORLD EXPERIMENTS TO CONFIRM YOUR IBS CAUSES

When I was sick with IBS and endometriosis, I kept searching for the one thing that would make everything better. I would research until I found something I hadn't tested yet—a supplement, a test, a food change—and try it. Each time, I was convinced that I would hit the jackpot and feel all better.

Maybe like you, I learned about many possible things that could help me. I learned about antimicrobial herbs, like berberine or neem, special diets, like the low FODMAP diet, and supplements like L-glutamine or Betaine HCl (stomach acid). But this was all in a disorganized soup, and I realized much too late that I didn't have any idea how or when to use these tools appropriately.

And once I started studying to become a nutrition professional, I fell even deeper into this rabbit hole. I was sure that I could help others find *their* magic pill.

The truth I've discovered, through my own struggles, and now supporting clients, is this: the missing secret to success for IBS isn't any particular magic pill, test, treatment, or diet.

Instead, it's the way you use those tools and how you investigate that helps you find your root causes and what's uniquely true for you.

The surprising thing that you need to heal yourself from the inside out is a strategy. A clear strategy will help you use the tools at your disposal properly for the best benefit.

Most IBS patients wade into the flood of possible options without much guidance about where to start or go next. If you've done things this way, don't feel ashamed. It's a natural outcome of the thousands of blogs, videos, and books out there that can easily overwhelm you.

Here are just some of the most common questions I've received from my subscribers and clients over the years that illustrate what this looks like for real people:

- Is coffee good or bad to drink when you have SIBO?
- Is it okay to consume alcohol when suffering from a leaky gut? What drinks are safe?
- Are organic yogurts and goat's milk okay if the gut heals and if there are no symptoms? I'm scared to test them in case I haven't healed or they secretly harm the gut.
- Which probiotics should I use for SIBO, and when should I use them? I heard I shouldn't use probiotics for SIBO, so who's right?
- I have low good bacteria and high bad bacteria. I'm trying the SCD diet, but I also have 66 food intolerances so I'm not left with much. Has anyone had any success with the SCD diet? My naturopath did a stool test and said it looks like SIBO.
- I've been tested for food sensitivities and don't have any (other than gluten and I've been gluten-free for eight years). Would you still keep a food diary? I've

been going at it for about a month and there have been no stand-out connections between foods and how good or bad my guts are.

- Has anyone here healed from SIBO? If so, how? What diet did you implement? What supplements did you take?
- Do I need to address SIFO and SIBO prior to probiotics? My microbiome is depleted of *Lactobacillus* probably because I'm dairy intolerant so I have been avoiding it.
- My doctor told me to do the FODMAP diet. I then later met with a GI doctor who told me that doctors should not put me on that diet since I have IBS-C, not IBS-D.
- I heard that I should eat whatever I want during SIBO treatment to feed the bacteria, and then go back to eating clean after, is this right?

You can clearly see that if you're confused about these kinds of questions, you're not alone.

You can't change the flood of confusing information, but you DO have the power to step off the merry-go-round now and commit to creating your custom IBS solution by using strategy.

In all honesty, I can guarantee that whatever you've researched so far to combat your bloating, pain, and irregular bowel movements is potentially a useful tool that you can use to find your unique IBS solution. But you need an additional key to help you find which of those options is best and right for YOU.

The way to answer questions like these is to become the Head Detective of your personal IBS journey by using a strategy I call the Iterative Action Method. Let me show you how I help my clients answer these questions, and really any question you could ask about your IBS.

A Method to the IBS Madness

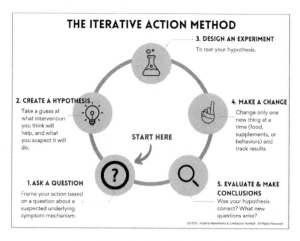

Figure 2: The Iterative Action Method.

The **Iterative Action Method** is a powerful framework I developed to help IBS patients use strategic experiments to find symptom relief. The word "**iterative**" simply means that you are learning by doing and building on what you learn. If you've ever taken a high school science class, you might be familiar with this approach as the scientific method. It's a process for answering questions that don't have easy answers.

Because IBS has many potential root causes, and not all of them are diagnosable by testing, the Iterative Action Method helps you use questioning and experimenting to illuminate some of the more elusive reasons for your signs and symptoms. Using this method, you can narrow down all the hundreds of potential IBS tools you've read about to the few specific options that will best help you improve your symptoms.

Let's explore the Iterative Action Method and how to use it.

Step 1: Ask a Question

To find the answers you're looking for, you'll first need to ask the right question.

Consider that every single thing you try, test, or change to help your IBS symptoms is asking one or both of *these two questions*:

- **Does this change (technique, treatment, medication, supplement, behavior change, diet, or food change) make my symptoms better or worse?**
- **What is the mechanism of that change? In other words, why does it do that?**

When you test something new through the lens of how and why it's affecting your symptoms, you're then able to see how to transform them.

For example, let's say you plan to try out a new probiotic supplement. What you're ultimately wondering is, do probiotics improve my IBS symptoms? But you want to take that question further and ask, "If so, what does that mean about my gut?"

So the question, therefore, will be:

"Is a bacterial imbalance one of the causes of my IBS symptoms?" because adding probiotic bacteria to your gut helps balance your gut microbiome. This is HOW it works.

As another example, say you're considering trying the low FODMAP diet (a diet low in fermentable carbohydrates). The question you're really asking with this experiment is:

"Do high FODMAP foods trigger my IBS symptoms?"

You can even apply this questioning method to medications that your doctor has prescribed. If your doctor prescribed Linzess for constipation, your question would be:

"Does the action mechanism of *Linzess* improve my constipation and gut motility?"

When you approach your experiments with this kind of question in mind, the outcome of those experiments will help you get clear answers about how your symptoms work, and this shows you what you need to know to begin managing them.

Step 2: Make a Hypothesis

Next, you'll predict what you think will happen when you add or change whatever you plan to test. It's helpful to tie your hypothesis to your specific symptoms and what you expect might happen.

Your hypothesis should predict a mechanism. In other words, consider why you think it will work.

Your statement, or hypothesis, could be:

"I think probiotics will reduce my constipation," or, "I think a low FODMAP diet will improve my bloating." Or, "I think a course of rifaximin (antibiotics) will improve my SIBO numbers and symptoms."

This hypothesis:

- Establishes a specific reaction that you hope to see.
- Helps you frame what you will be tracking.
- Will help you decide whether your experiment was a success or not.

Step 3: Design a Test or Experiment

Now, you'll design an experiment to test your theory, just like with your science fair project in school; except, this time, you are the study subject!

One of the most important concepts to master when designing an experiment is to *only test one new thing at a time.*

A common pitfall for IBS patients trying to feel better is to layer on many new things at once, such as diets, supplements, and routine changes. It's understandable and even admirable that you want to take decisive action! But when you change too many things at once, you won't get clear answers to your questions because you won't be sure what caused the changes you observed. Was it the increase in chewing? The digestive enzyme tablets? The antibiotics?

So design an experiment that tests only one variable at a time.

Choose just one tool, technique, or protocol for your experiment. Everything from diet changes, medications, supplements, behavior changes, or therapies are your experiment choices.

Here are some examples of tests or experiments you could choose to get more clarity about the causes of your IBS symptoms:

- Try an elimination diet like the low FODMAP diet.
- Eliminate a single, suspected problem food for two to three weeks.
- Use rifaximin and neomycin antibiotic treatment for SIBO for 14 to 21 days.
- Practice meditation daily for two weeks.
- Chew each bite of food 25 times at every meal for a week.
- Try digestive enzymes for 30 days.

Create a clear time frame that you plan to test, and make appropriate preparations for your experiment, if necessary.

Step 4: Run Your Experiment

Now, it's time to make the specific changes you've planned.

Make daily observations about how your symptoms change or shift during your experiment. Of course, one of the most important things to track is if and how your bowel movements or other IBS symptoms are changing.

One of my favorite tracking methods I recommend for clients is a Food, Mood, and Poop journal, which my mentor and teacher, Andrea Nakayama of The Functional Nutrition Alliance created. (See a complete discussion about the Food, Mood, Poop journal in Chapter 4.) Using this tool, you track what you eat, your signs and symptoms ("mood"), and your bowel movements. You can also track your symptoms in any way that makes sense for you.

If your experiment is long, you can track your symptoms for a few days in the beginning and then again at the end of your experiment.

At this stage, I only want you to make observations, not conclusions. Just take notes and data over the course of the experiment.

Step 5: Evaluate Results and Make Conclusions

Now that you've completed your experiment, it's time to evaluate what happened and draw some conclusions. The main question you want to ask yourself at this stage is:

"Did the change make me feel better, the same, or worse?"

By working alongside the observations you made in your Food, Mood, Poop journal or other tracking systems, you should be able to objectively evaluate whether you saw any kind of improvement, no change at all, or a worsening of symptoms.

If your symptoms improved, this tells you that whatever mechanism you were testing is one of your IBS root causes.

So, for example, if you had less cramping and diarrhea after eliminating dairy products from your diet, this suggests that either lactose intolerance (milk sugar) or casein sensitivity (dairy protein) is a mechanism of your symptoms.

Suppose completing the elimination phase of the low FODMAP diet (more on this in Chapter 4) improved your bloating and constipation. In that case, this means that your digestive system is intolerant to certain fermentable foods and that excess bacteria are likely doing the fermenting.

If your symptoms stayed the same, then this tells you that the mechanism you were testing with your experiment has nothing to do with your symptoms. Though this may feel like a waste of time, it's actually a win because you now know you can stop spending energy on actions that address that symptom mechanism.

For example, if completing the elimination phase of the low FODMAP diet didn't change anything for the better or worse, this tells you that fermentable carbohydrates are unrelated to your symptoms. With this key information, you can now test a different possible food-symptom mechanism or other treatment option.

If your symptoms got worse, then this tells you that something about your experiment is related to your underlying symptom mechanisms. This is also crucial information for you to help you make the right treatment decisions.

For example, if taking probiotics before meals has only worsened your constipation, this might tell you that you likely already have too much bacteria in your gut or that you don't tolerate prebiotic ingredients in the probiotics. In turn, this suggests you may need to focus on reducing bacteria in your gut.

Now that you have made this conclusion, you can move along and consider what your next steps should be. **And here is an extremely important detail: your next steps will be based on what you learned in this round of Iterative Action!**

Many people in the IBS space will lay out complex roadmaps that say, "First, you'll do this diet, then you'll start this supplement, and then you'll do this treatment," and so on. I don't find these roadmaps useful because they don't take into account how things have changed with the first step. What happens at stage one should determine your next steps, not an arbitrary, theoretical recipe.

The outcome of each experiment you complete will be what you rely on to choose your next steps. This way, you continually refine your approach to be more responsive and customized to what your body is actually telling you.

So if your symptoms improved from your experiment, you'd choose another possible symptom mechanism to test that might help resolve your remaining symptoms. If your symptoms stayed the same, you'd create a new question, hypothesis, and experiment to test a different possible symptom mechanism.

And suppose your symptoms got worse from your experiment. In that case, you'll use that information to consider what might be responsible for that mechanism and design a new experiment to test your new theory.

The point is to use what you've learned so far and build on that knowledge to fill in missing information gaps. In this way, you create a unique collection of tools that you know, by direct experience, truly help you feel better and address your particular underlying symptom mechanisms. There is no better medicine.

To give you a better example of what this looks like in real life, I'd like to share with you three interesting case studies from my clients that demonstrate the power of The Iterative Action Method to resolve IBS symptoms. I have changed my clients' names to protect their privacy.

Case Study: Jack and His Food Sensitivities

Jack is a happy, energetic 30-something man who has had chronic IBS-D for over ten years. He has many food sensitivities that make eating out difficult. And if he veers at all from his narrow diet template, he notices an increase in diarrhea.

When Jack started my Calm Digestion Method program, he felt clearly that stress was a significant contributor to his symptoms. So he started with stress relief foundations (see Chapter 3) and saw some amazing progress in well-being just by chewing and feeling grateful at meals. So he's incorporated these practices into his regular routine. However, he still couldn't waver from his restrictive diet (see Chapter 4).

Jack's next hypothesis was that infections were contributing to his long-term food sensitivities. We ran a GI MAP stool test, which showed an *H. pylori* infection and two parasites that none of his doctors had previously identified. We also ran a SIBO test, which was negative.

At this stage, his main question is whether or not *H. pylori* is a significant contributor to his symptoms. He tested a treatment protocol to see if and how his symptoms change. His next steps will depend on the answers he learns from this trial.

Case Study: Dave and Chronic Hemorrhoids

Dave is a middle-aged man who had had severe constipation for many years when he met me. This chronic constipation had led to severe hemorrhoids, which required surgery. The surgery had not resolved them.

Dave had worked with multiple practitioners including an acupuncturist, a primary care doctor, and a gastroenterologist. He had also made some diet changes and experimented with a few supplements, but he still wasn't sure what to do.

By applying the Iterative Action Method strategic approach, Dave considered what he already knew and where his knowledge gaps were. His first question was whether or not he might be eating foods that were worsening his constipation.

When we reviewed what he already knew about which foods were a problem for him, they almost perfectly aligned with the list of high FODMAP foods. So Dave asked the question, "Are FODMAP foods making my constipation worse?" Dave did a low FODMAP elimination diet for a few weeks and found that his constipation was a little better. So he learned that FODMAP foods were indeed related to his symptoms. Some food reintroduction experiments confirmed his specific sensitivities.

However, the diet didn't completely resolve his symptoms, and he was still struggling with straining and hemorrhoids. Dave was curious if there had been any missed infections that might be causing a problem. He decided to run a GI MAP stool test and a SIBO breath test.

Testing revealed an *H. pylori* infection and a parasite, so his question became, "Are my digestive symptoms being caused by my *H. pylori* infection?" Almost immediately after Dave began his treatment, his bowel movements significantly improved. By the time he finished his 14-day regimen, he felt better than he had in years. He concluded that his *H. pylori* infection was somehow impacting his constipation, which was then causing hemorrhoids.

This case shows the power of using the Iterative Action Method to methodically choose action steps and the power of working at the most likely upstream cause.

Case Study: John and His Chronic IBS-D

When John first entered my program, he had had IBS-D for over ten years. If he used activated charcoal daily, he could function alright. But his bowels kept him largely in the house, and he avoided social outings in case he couldn't find a bathroom. John had had scopes done that didn't show anything useful.

In addition to considering what he already knew about what made his symptoms better or worse and how they first started, John tested his stool with a GI MAP and completed a SIBO breath test.

John's SIBO test was clearly positive. His GI MAP showed some mild dysbiosis, and a possible gluten sensitivity, but didn't show any sign of IBD or pancreatic insufficiency.

John's first Iterative Action Experiment was to ask whether gluten was increasing his symptoms. He decided to try reducing gluten to see if that made any difference while he waited to consult with his doctor about further treatment. He felt his symptoms improved a little, but nowhere near the improvement he was looking for.

His GP prescribed a SIBO treatment, which he tried next. His question here was whether SIBO was causing his diarrhea symptoms. After about five days of treatment, John had his first solid bowel movement without supplements in many years. He was ecstatic! And he had an answer to his question.

A few weeks after his SIBO treatment, his symptoms returned, this time worse than ever. This often happens after treatment, and can suggest that the change in the microbiome from the antibiotics allowed another resident to become dominant, like *C. difficile* or *Candida*, or it can often suggest that SIBO is still present. After consulting with his GP, he tested for *C. difficile*, which was negative. So he decided to try treating for

SIBO again, a little more aggressively, since this was what had worked before.

By the end of his protocol, he was once again feeling well; a few months later, John could go out in the world and do work he loves again because he's not always needing a bathroom.

John's process illustrates the Iterative Action Method perfectly: ask good questions, complete experiments based on your hypothesis, evaluate what happened, rely on what you learned to make good decisions, and act accordingly. Using this process, he found his way to lasting symptom relief.

Successful IBS Treatment Depends on Your Strategy

In this chapter, you've come to understand that through the Iterative Action Method, you can figure out, one clue at a time, what's causing your IBS symptoms. And the most important skill you can cultivate as an IBS patient is to structure your experiments and tests in a methodical way so that they build on each other, step-by-step.

What's so special about this method is that it's never too late to begin. Whether you've been sitting with this discomfort and frustration for years or it has just recently appeared, you can use this method to organize your ideas and find your path to IBS symptom resolution.

So I invite you to commit to using the Iterative Action Method to explore the underlying causes of your symptoms and to engage with your food, supplement, medication, or behavior experiments to learn more about why your symptoms are happening.

In the next four chapters, I'll be sharing the most research-backed Iterative Action Experiments to use in your quest to relieve your IBS symptoms. The Iterative Action Method will be a guiding star in these chapters.

3

STRESS: THE ELEPHANT IN THE BATHROOM

No conversation about digestion can be complete without discussing stress.

Stress, big and small, fills our 21st-century lives. In prehistoric times, humans likely experienced stress in short bursts and recovered quickly, when today this exception has become the rule. For many of us, feeling stressed is as natural as breathing.

So how does stress affect your digestive system?

Quite dramatically, it turns out. Though it's not often the *only* underlying cause of your IBS symptoms, stress uniquely affects your digestion and needs to be tamed. Many IBS patients find from their assessment process that stressful events were a significant symptom trigger or that stress is a common symptom mediator.

In this chapter, I'm going to explain the profound effects stress has on the digestive system, and explain how some simple, daily practices can help improve your mood, energy, and, most importantly, your digestive symptoms.

The Gut-Brain Connection

Under moments of stress, whether from the imminent threat of death or the thought of traffic making you late for work, your nervous system changes its priorities.

Most of us think of stress as coming from the brain. Would it surprise you to know that stress is more of a whole-body effect and closely tied to your digestive system?

If you've ever experienced "butterflies in your stomach" when you were excited or anxious about an upcoming event, you've witnessed the "gut-brain connection" in action.

When you feel relaxed, your nervous system is in the "rest-and-digest" state. In this state, your **parasympathetic nervous system** is activated. When you're happy, with your favorite people, enjoying yourself, or doing the things you love, you're in the rest-and-digest state.

Your digestion is designed to work when you are in the rest-and-digest state.

When you're experiencing stress, your nervous system switches to what's called the **fight-flight-or-freeze response.** Any kind of stress, big or small, can lead to this switch. Someone cutting you off in traffic, a critical remark from your spouse, or being late for work are small examples, while losing a loved one, getting fired, or feeling very stressed about money could be examples of larger modern-day stresses. In addition, the ongoing stress of being sick with a chronic illness like IBS and feeling hopeless is its own unique stress.

When you're in this fight-flight-or-freeze state, your body is priming itself to run away from a threat or stand and fight. To do this, it directs your body to release adrenaline, which gives you extra energy. And crucially for our conversation, this stress leads your body to direct blood away from your digestive system and reproductive organs and sends it to your muscles, heart, and lungs.

In other words, *it literally slows or stops your digestion to prepare you for a fight or a flight.*

Ongoing and chronic micro-stresses will repeatedly shift your body into the fight-flight-or-freeze state and disrupt your digestion. If you've noticed that stress makes your IBS symptoms worse, this is a strong indicator that it will be essential for you to find ways to tame that stress to improve your condition.

Trauma and IBS

Traumatic events in your past can create a special kind of fight-flight-or-freeze state that can significantly impact your immune and digestive systems, and these deserve special mention.

Adverse childhood experiences (ACEs), such as abuse, loss, or having substance-abusing caregivers or partners, can generate lifelong nervous system changes, leading to chronic activation of the fight-or-flight response.

People who experienced ACEs are much more likely to have autoimmune diseases, digestive disorders, cardiac disease, and many other kinds of health problems throughout their lifetime (Dube et. al., 2009; Sonu et. al., 2019). Your body responds similarly if you're an adult when the trauma occurs.

American author and psychiatrist Bessel Van der Kolk explores the consequences of trauma in his 2015 book *The Body Keeps the Score: Brain, Mind, and Body in the Healing of Trauma.*

He writes:

"While we all want to move beyond trauma, the part of our brain that is devoted to ensuring our survival (deep below our rational brain) is not very good at denial. Long after a traumatic experience is over, it may be reactivated at the slightest hint of danger and mobilize disturbed brain circuits, and secrete massive amounts of stress hormone."

This kind of trauma response can often and easily trigger IBS symptoms, including food reactions, panic attacks, diarrhea, cramps, and other physical pain sensations. Sometimes, rewiring this kind of trauma response is an essential step to overcoming IBS.

IF YOU FOUND THAT STRESS WAS A SIGNIFICANT PART OF YOUR IBS triggers or mediators, let's look at the Iterative Action Experiments you can try to find relief from IBS symptoms.

Iterative Action Experiments to Find Your Personal Stress Remedy

It's highly likely that stress in some way, shape, or form is connected to your IBS symptoms. Because the stress response literally slows or stops your digestive function, it's imperative to meet this challenge head-on. I highly recommend addressing stress as one of your first foundational Iterative Action Experiments.

Reducing stress is one of the simplest ways to enhance your digestive function. Though it may seem inconsequential, paying attention to this first foundation of gut health can profoundly affect your overall healing process.

What follows is a collection of options you can try to see what makes the most difference for your IBS symptoms. As with any list of IBS remedies, not all of these will be relevant for you.

Remember to use the Iterative Action Method with each change you make, asking a clear question you hope to answer, creating a hypothesis that explains what you expect, designing an experiment, tracking your results, and making some conclusions. As always, try only one new thing at a time to get the best feedback about whether or not it is truly effective for you. Refer back to Chapter 2 if you need help setting up your experiment.

Mealtime Zen

When you eat your meals, how is your mood? Do you eat in a rush? Do you even stop to eat? Do you feel anxious about what food is going to do to your digestion?

If you answered 'yes' to any of these questions, you might want to experiment with your eating habits. In many cases, creating relaxation habits around your meal times can keep your nervous system in the rest-and-digest state and have a surprising effect on your IBS symptoms.

Creating an enjoyable, stress-free experience at every mealtime prepares your gut to properly digest your food, while eating in a stressed-out mood sets you up for indigestion and symptoms.

Here are some suggested eating habits to create mealtime Zen.

Prepare Yourself for Eating

Prepare to eat by taking a few deep breaths and appreciating the aroma and visual presentation of your food. This meditative practice brings your nervous system into rest-and-digest and prepares you for enjoyment. It also encourages your body to begin secreting vital digestive juices like stomach acid, saliva, and digestive enzymes, which are essential for good digestion.

If you often feel anxious about what effect food will have on your digestion, practice reciting an affirmation or mantra to reinforce the positive things that food does for you. For example, "I trust that this food will nourish me and digest well."

Chewing

Chewing is a significant part of digestion. It mechanically breaks down your food and mixes it with saliva, which helps begin the digestion of your carbohydrates. **Because carbohydrates are often troublesome foods for IBS patients, this practice is especially important.**

In addition, settling into the habit of chewing can be a meditation. I often think of my field cow, Phoebe, and how relaxed she is when she's lying in the sun chewing her cud. She's not thinking about what she'll be doing after lunch or where she has to be. She's simply present and relaxed, chewing.

So aim to spend time chewing each and every bite of your food. While you're chewing, appreciate the flavors and textures you're experiencing. Be present in the moment. Try putting your fork down in between bites. **A minimum goal would be twenty chews per bite.**

Liquid Intake at Meals

Drinking liquids during your meal can dilute the digestive juices your gut relies on to digest your food well.

To prevent this, avoid drinking large amounts of water from 30 minutes before until one hour after eating. Drinking a little while you eat is alright, but don't chug a huge glass of water, soda, alcohol, or other liquids with your meal.

Meditation & Breathing for IBS Relief

It's a well-documented fact that meditation or breathing practices provide many kinds of health benefits to those that use them regularly. There is also good evidence suggesting that these types of practices directly help IBS patients feel better.

I think meditation and breathing are one of the best options to address the pervasive micro-stresses we experience in modern life. No matter how much we try, we'll likely continue to feel stressed about things daily.

So just like doing physical activity like walking or biking daily helps us to stay healthy, meditation or breathing exercise should be viewed as a recommended daily practice. This helps to remind your nervous system how to access the rest-and-digest state easily.

There are a variety of meditation options that can help you improve your stress levels, resilience, and IBS symptoms. Use the Iterative Action Method to test one or more that resonate with you to find what most helps you relieve your stress and your associated IBS symptoms. Here are some ideas.

- **Find a local meditation class or teacher** to support you in practicing mindfulness and meditation. A retreat might be a good jumpstart option. You could also try online classes.
- **Brain balancing sound technology meditation recordings,** like EquiSync, are great for daily meditation. These tracks exercise different types of brain waves, and only take 23 minutes per day. (See Resources.)
- **Meditation apps**, like HeadSpace and Calm provide guided meditations, soothing music, daily check-ins, and more to help you practice stress relief.

- **Self-hypnosis apps or videos** available for free online can also help restore balance to your brain if used regularly.

With some dedicated attention to keeping your nervous system calm and centered, I'm confident you'll experience fewer IBS symptoms. You may also find other benefits.

Physical Activity

We know that physical exercise helps keep us healthy and that it also helps release endorphins (feel-good chemicals). It turns out it also has benefits for our digestive system.

Physical movement can literally get our bowels moving and help excess gas escape. So especially if you're constipated or are generally sedentary, trying an Iterative Action Experiment to increase daily physical activity might improve your IBS symptoms.

Yoga, Pilates, swimming, biking, walking, or anything you enjoy will help you keep your digestive processes working smoothly.

Retraining an Overactive or Traumatized Nervous System

For those of you with highly-reactive nervous systems, or a background with trauma, this can be a strong indicator that your nervous system needs significant attention. If this is true for you, it will likely be challenging for you to make headway with your symptoms until this is appropriately addressed.

Read through the following list of symptoms that suggest your brain and nervous system are on high alert:

- You feel like you're in a constant state of anxiety and vigilance.
- Every little setback feels like a catastrophe.
- Negative emotions frequently trigger you.
- You have a high level of reactions to food, supplements, chemicals, or even water...no matter what you put into your body, you react.
- You have difficulty falling asleep or staying in REM sleep.
- You startle easily.

If this sounds like you, your first Iterative Action Experiment priority should be to work on rehabilitating your nervous system. You may not be able to benefit from any other methods, techniques, or treatments if your nervous system is in a hyper-reactive state.

Here are some great possible ways to help you retrain your nervous system. See which one feels most right to you, and design an Iterative Action Experiment to test it. (See the Resources Section for more information about accessing these options.)

Dynamic Neural Retraining System (DNRS)

Designed and developed by Annie Hopper, DNRS is a self-directed online program that helps rewire your brain and calm the fight-flight-or-freeze response.

Gupta Program

Designed and developed by Ashok Gupta, this self-directed online program supports you in creating a daily meditation practice and retraining the amygdala, or the fear center of the brain, with a specialized Amygdala Retraining Technique (ART).

Eye Movement and Desensitization Reprocessing (EMDR)

EMDR is a specialized type of psychotherapy designed to help resolve trauma and Post-Traumatic Stress Disorder (PTSD). A trained therapist uses sound, lights, or hand buzzers to bring traumatic memories to the surface so you can process them with the safety of a therapist.

Emotional Freedom Technique (EFT)

Emotional Freedom Technique uses a series of "tapping" on specific body points to help process traumatic memories. It has shown benefits for PTSD. A trained practitioner or therapist usually facilitates the process.

It doesn't really matter which of these stress relief options you choose, so long as they are effective for you. Choose the option that most resonates with you, and get busy applying the Iterative Action Method to explore which options help relieve your IBS symptoms.

Your goal is to find your unique combination of stress relief and eating habits that most reduces your IBS symptoms. It will be unique for each reader.

When you find something that works, continue using the technique as one of your keystone action steps, and look back at your list of likely root causes to choose your next Iterative Action Experiment.

Now that we've covered stress, let's move on to managing your food choices with proper diet experimentation.

4

WHAT THE HECK SHOULD YOU BE EATING FOR IBS?

Food is one of the first areas I recommend focusing your Iterative Action Experiments on after stress relief. Most people eat food daily, so if you're continuously eating foods that are flaring your IBS, this is obviously fanning the flames of your symptoms. The trouble is, what should you be eating?

If you're not sure, you're not alone. One of the most common struggles I hear about from my IBS and SIBO clients is confusion and uncertainty about what they should or shouldn't be eating.

And with the help of Dr. Google, some people start limiting their diet further and further until their eating list is just down to a few foods. Or they start trying out all the diets they've read about, while getting more confused. Some people doggedly keep to an unnecessary diet for far longer than they should.

Though many people crave a cookie-cutter diet solution, there just isn't one when it comes to food. Each of you will be unique. You can use diet templates to guide you, but each and every one will need to be adapted for you to be used appropriately.

A good example is one of my clients who stayed on the Candida diet for *eight years* even though it wasn't showing any clear benefit.

Some days it can feel like you understand what your gut reacts to. Then, when you least expect it, something you've come to trust betrays you. Or maybe your symptoms remain the same no matter what you try to change. *Why?*

The answer comes back to the central question we asked in Chapter 1, "What's causing your IBS?" And the key question to answer when trying to figure out what to eat to control your IBS symptoms is what MECHANISM is causing your food symptoms. Is it a FODMAP sensitivity? Lactose intolerance? Trouble with dietary histamines? Again, it comes down to asking questions that will show you *how* your symptoms are happening.

When you approach your dietary changes from this perspective and use the Iterative Action Method to run your experiments, you get increasingly useful information about what mechanism is responsible for triggering your food-related gut symptoms. And then, rather than relying on conflicting lists of foods you should eat or avoid, you can create your own customized list that is specifically tailored to the unique causes of your food-related IBS symptoms.

To get started, let's talk about the proper way to make dietary changes.

The Correct Way to Use A Therapeutic IBS Diet

Specialized diets are useful tools for helping control physical signs and symptoms. But used improperly, they can become restrictive, challenging to maintain, and, worst of all, can lead to malnutrition.

I've met many clients who have driven themselves nearly crazy trying to maintain a restrictive diet, much to the chagrin of their families. Most people, left to their own devices with the internet or books, forge ahead with the best intentions, but use these diets incorrectly.

So let me first explain the correct way to use a therapeutic —also known as an elimination—diet.

The first thing I want to ensure you know is that **any diet change that you'll be making is fundamentally an Iterative Action Experiment.** You'll be designing that experiment to answer a question you have about whether that food, or the underlying mechanism of that group of foods, is responsible for your symptoms.

For example, if you're trying a low FODMAP diet, you're testing the mechanism of fermentable carbohydrates as a potential symptom cause. If you're removing dairy, you're testing the mechanism of lactose (dairy sugar) or casein (dairy protein) as the source of your symptoms.

Getting clear on this helps you get the best data out of your food experiments. If a food category causes symptoms, then avoid it as needed. *If not, you're barking up the wrong tree, and you don't have to keep avoiding those foods!*

The basic therapeutic elimination diet experiment has three phases:

1. **Elimination Phase:** *During this phase, you eliminate a food—or foods—you suspect of being a symptom trigger.* Usually, the elimination phase should last 2-3 weeks at the maximum, as this is usually long enough to see a positive or negative (or no change) result from the experiment. Remember, your job here is to determine if your hypothesis about the mechanism you're testing is correct or not.

2. **Reintroduction Phase:** *If the elimination phase improved your symptoms, now you'll carefully reintroduce the foods you removed, one at a time, to test for clear reactions.* It's often the case that not *all* of the foods you removed cause reactions. The more clarity you get here, the fewer foods you have to restrict long term.

3. **Maintenance Phase:** *Using what you've learned from the elimination and reintroduction phases, you create a food plan* that avoids foods that cause symptoms and includes foods that don't trigger symptoms.

Additionally, food reintroductions can be confusing, so here are a few tips to support you.

A FEW TIPS FOR FOOD REINTRODUCTIONS

1. The elimination phase of any diet is not meant to be used as your long-term diet template. Once you find the elimination phase improves your symptoms, move right on to doing reintroductions.

2. When you reintroduce a food, if you feel fine and don't notice any symptoms, good! That means you can handle that food.

3. If you experience increased bloating, gas, pain, or stool changes, you'll want to avoid that food while you heal your gut.

4. Allow your digestive system to calm down after a reaction before you move on to testing another food item.

If you stick to this three-step process and focus on doing

Iterative Action Experiments with clear questions you're trying to answer, you *will* get clarity about which foods, or types of foods, are triggering your symptoms.

I like to say that knowing which foods are causing your symptoms is liberating. Knowing exactly what you can eat and what you need to avoid gives you the freedom to move about in the world knowing how to minimize your symptoms.

How to Choose Iterative Action Diet Experiments for IBS and SIBO

One of the hardest questions my IBS and SIBO clients struggle with is deciding which diet changes they should choose. And with good reason, because there are so many conflicting opinions about this.

Remember, your goal with food is to try to learn *how* they are causing symptoms, and you're going to use your food experiment to try and answer that question.

The way I like to help clients do this is to start with what they know. What do I mean by this? Well, rather than try a diet because somebody else says it should help, I have them make a list of foods **they already know make their symptoms worse**. Even if they're generally confused, most clients have a short list of foods they *know* they need to avoid to prevent symptoms.

I then have them compare their list with exclusion lists from the Low FODMAP diet, the low histamine diet, the low oxalate diet, or other therapeutic diets. (See later in this chapter for key lists for these diets. If you really don't know what foods make your symptoms better or worse, see the section later in this chapter titled "What If You Don't Know Which Foods Are Bothering You Yet?").

The majority of the time, I find that either FODMAP foods (fermentable carbohydrates) or high histamine foods are the primary mechanism for IBS symptoms. However, there are many other possibilities. You will have to figure out your unique food-symptom mechanism to make progress with your IBS symptoms.

Once you think you see a pattern in your list, then you can design an Iterative Action Experiment to test your theory. If you're right, great, now you have important information about how to control your symptoms. If you're wrong, you can make a new hypothesis, test that out, and so on.

Keep in mind that it may be possible that your symptoms have nothing to do with food at all. If, no matter what kind of changes you make to your diet, you don't see any symptom changes, this suggests you'll want to focus your efforts on other possible underlying causes.

So what follows in the rest of this chapter are diets that can be used as Iterative Action Experiments to help you discover your unique food-symptom mechanism so that you can control your food-related IBS symptoms. I've done my best to provide the necessary context you need to help reduce your food confusion and help you understand what to eat and what not to eat. However, you may need professional help to best navigate these diet changes, so don't be afraid to reach out to a qualified coach or professional if you need help.

Quick Gut Reset Experiment

A quick gut reset can be a way to rapidly relieve symptoms of IBS and SIBO, especially if your symptoms are constantly flaring. This is a wonderful way to prepare a "clean canvas" for more expert and complex elimination diets used afterward. Gut expert Dr. Michael Ruscio recommends this technique in his book *Healthy Gut, Healthy You.*

There are two ways you can go about doing a quick gut reset:

1. **Dr. Ruscio's *Elemental Heal* product** is a liquid meal replacement that starves the bacteria that may be contributing to bloating, pain, diarrhea, or constipation. You can choose between the regular, dairy-free, or low-carb options. You'll replace all your meals for three days with Elemental Heal and keep tabs on whether your symptoms improve. Use Dr. Ruscio's dosing calculator to decide how much product to buy for the three days. See the Resources section for where to find Elemental Heal and the Dosing Calculator.

2. **A 3-Day Bone Broth Fast** can be a helpful way to reduce bloating, pain, constipation, or diarrhea, by removing all fiber that may cause symptoms, but without complete fasting. Simple bone broth also contains gut-healing nutrients, like glycine and collagen, that can help repair your gut lining. If you know you're sensitive to histamine, a bone broth fast is probably not a good idea, as bone broth can be high in histamine.

If you see dramatic, positive results from this 3-day reset, this tells you that fiber is likely one of the mechanisms contributing to your symptoms, as this reset removes all fiber and reduces your diet to the basic nutrition building blocks. Now let's explore the low FODMAP diet.

The Low FODMAP Diet Experiment

The therapeutic diet with the clearest data about its benefit for IBS patients is the low FODMAP diet (Zahedi et. al. 2018; Gibson et. al., 2010; Gibson, 2017; Pederson et. al., 2017; Zhan et. al., 2018; Cox et. al., 2020). For this reason, if your list of things that make your symptoms worse in your assessment includes multiple high FODMAP foods, or if you haven't done any work with your diet yet, this is one of the first dietary Iterative Action Experiments I recommend for those with IBS.

FODMAP stands for Fermentable Oligosaccharides, Disaccharides, Monosaccharides, and Polyols, which are fancy words for different types of natural sugars and carbohydrates found in foods. Therefore, a Low FODMAP diet involves removing these fermentable sugars and starches from your food plan for a while.

There are six types of specific FODMAPS: Fructose, Lactose, Mannitol, Sorbitol, Galacto-oligosaccharides, and Fructans. These six fermentable carbohydrates occur naturally in whole foods, such as vegetables, fruits, dairy products, or nuts. You can be sensitive to one, a few, or all of these types of carbohydrates.

Though the foods on a high FODMAP list are generally considered healthy, their fiber or sugar content provides food for any excess bacteria in your digestive system. If you're sensitive to FODMAP foods, you may experience bloating, distention, abdominal pain, constipation, or diarrhea when you eat them.

Here is a partial list of high-FODMAP foods:

Vegetables & Fruits	Nuts, Grains, & Legumes	Dairy, Sweeteners, & Miscellaneous
Broccoli	Almonds	Milk
Cauliflower	Cashews	Cheese
Cabbage	Pistachios	Ice cream
Brussels sprouts	(Other nuts ok, in serving size	Yogurt
Collard greens	of 10 nuts)	Sugar alcohols (xylitol,
Onions	Wheat (Gluten)	sorbitol,
Garlic	Barley	erythritol)
Celery	Rye	High-fructose corn syrup
Mushrooms	Beans	Agave syrup
Beets	Lentils	Honey
Peas	Chickpeas/Garbanzo beans	Fruit juice concentrate
Artichoke		Inulin
Asparagus		FOS/GOS (Prebiotics)
Corn		Chicory
Apples		
Pears		
Plums		
Apricots		
Nectarines		
Peaches		
Avocado		
Blackberries		
Blueberries		
Cherries		
Dates		
Figs		
Mango		
Dried fruit		
Fruit juice		

Table 4: Partial list of common high FODMAP foods.

The definitive resource for understanding the specific levels of FODMAPs in foods is the Monash University app. Available on the App Store, you can use Monash to explore which foods contain FODMAPs as well as which specific types of FODMAPs are present in foods.

To test the hypothesis of whether high FODMAP foods are part of your symptom mechanism, you'll do a 2-3 week elimination diet, where you remove high FODMAP foods as much as possible and see what happens.

If you feel better during this elimination period, you've discovered that FODMAPs are one of your food-symptom triggers.

Once you know FODMAPs are your mechanism, your next Iterative Action Experiment will be to reintroduce FODMAP foods to figure out which specific types of FODMAPs are your personal kryptonite. Typically, you aren't sensitive to all FODMAP categories or foods.

I always like to remind my clients that FODMAPs are a sensitivity of quantity and frequency, meaning that your goal is to figure out how much FODMAP food you can eat and how often but not have symptoms. You won't ever be able to eat a zero FODMAP diet, and you shouldn't need to.

There are specific foods you can use to test each category of FODMAPs. So your first follow-up experiment will be to test each group, one at a time, using one of the recommended test foods. See the table below for specifics.

FODMAP group	Foods to test group
Fructose	4 sun-dried tomatoes, ¼ cup mango, OR 1 cup artichoke hearts
Lactose	3 tablespoons plain cow milk yogurt, ¼ cup whole milk, OR ¼ cup cream
Mannitol	⅓ medium stalk celery, ¾ cup cauliflower, OR ⅔ cup sweet potato
Sorbitol	¼ whole avocado, ⅓ cup yellow peach, OR ¼ of 1 medium green bell pepper
Galacto-oligosaccharides	¼ cup canned black beans, ⅛ cup green peas, OR 15 almonds
Fructan	½ leek, ½ cup zucchini, OR 1 clove garlic

Table 5: FODMAP reintroduction test foods and quantities. Source: Vital Food Therapeutics. Used with permission.

ONCE YOU KNOW WHICH GROUP OR GROUPS ARE YOUR PROBLEM, you can get more granular with each group.

For example, let's say you discovered that you, like many people with IBS, are sensitive to galacto-oligosaccharides, and you discovered this because you reacted when you tried eating green peas. But you went on to test a variety of legumes and found that black beans and edamame don't bother you, but garbanzo beans and kidney beans will really make you gassy. In addition, you learned that if you ate just a few kidney beans on a salad, you were fine, but if you ate a whole bowl of chili, you were in for a world of hurt.

Once you've done your reintroduction experiments and have clarity on which FODMAP foods do and don't work for you, you can now create a normal menu for yourself that honors your unique food sensitivities and helps minimize symptom flares. Win!

Using the FoodMarble AIRE 2 to Understand Your FODMAP Sensitivities

The FoodMarble AIRE 2 is a handheld home breath gas reader. The AIRE2 can be used to test for SIBO, but you can also use it to test for four FODMAP sensitivities, specifically lactose, fructose, sorbitol, and inulin. By drinking a challenge solution and then taking a gas reading with the AIRE 2 to check for a rise in hydrogen or methane gas, you can get specific information about whether you are sensitive to particular FODMAPs.

Using the AIRE 2 would work best after you've done a FODMAP elimination diet, but you could also use this tool to get that information quickly by doing this first. This would help you assess which groups of FODMAPs you're sensitive to right away, but you could still do individual food reintroductions to get more specific.

See the Resources section for information about ordering a FoodMarble AIRE 2.

The Low Fermentation Diet Experiment

Dr. Mark Pimentel and Dr. Ali Rezaie have created a new dietary theory—Low Fermentation Eating—that they described in their 2022 book *The Microbiome Connection*. This diet removes foods that they have observed most commonly cause fermentation, and therefore gas, in their IBS and SIBO patients' guts. This is the diet that they recommend to SIBO patients in their clinic.

The low fermentation diet is less restrictive than the low FODMAP diet and allows many foods considered high FODMAP. Though this initially surprised me, it's a good reminder that oftentimes people restrict their diet far beyond what's necessary.

This diet focuses on removing the most common causes of gas and fermentation and recommends spacing your meals at least four hours apart so that your gut is more likely to produce its normal natural cleaning waves between meals.

Here is a partial list of foods you can and can't eat on the low-fermentation diet plan:

Groups	What you can eat	What you cannot eat
Vegetables	Most other veggies, including small amounts of onions and garlic (cooked is best)	All cruciferous vegetables, artichoke, asparagus, alfalfa sprouts, bean sprouts, bok choy, chicory root, edamame, radish, snow peas, and sugar snap peas
Fruits	Most other fruits, one serving at a time.	Apples, dried fruit, bananas, dates, figs, fruit-juice concentrates, monk fruit, pears, prunes, and raisins
Proteins	All proteins	Commercial marinades
Grains	Simple carbohydrates like white bread, white rice, white pasta, cream of wheat, cornmeal, gnocchi, and tortilla chips	Bran, whole grain bread, brown rice, buckwheat flour, bulgar, whole wheat cereal, farrow, multigrain flour, oat bran, whole wheat pasta, soba noodles, and spelt flour
Nuts	Most all nuts	Chia seeds, flax seeds
Beans and legumes	N/A	Most beans and legumes
Dairy	Butter (small amounts), aged and hard cheese like parmesan & cheddar, alternative dairy milks, ghee, lactose-free cottage cheese, and lactose-free milk	Soft cheeses, cream cheese, milk, soy milk, yogurt. Avoid cultured lactose-free dairy products due to bacterial cultures.
Sweeteners	Cane sugar, maple syrup, and honey (small amounts)	Agave, erythritol, high fructose corn syrup, mannitol, monk fruit extract, saccharin, sorbitol, Splenda, stevia, sucralose, and xylitol

Table 6: A partial list of foods to eat and avoid on the Low Fermentation Eating plan. Source: Dr. Mark Pimentel and Dr. Ali Rezaie. Used with permission.

This diet especially suggests avoiding indigestible and fermentable fibers. You can find these fibers listed on food labels as inulin, oligofructose, oligofructose-enriched inulin, chicory root fiber, chicory root extract, and fructo-oligosaccharides. Manufacturers commonly add these thickeners or other additives to foods like yogurt, soups, coffee substitutes, candy, keto foods, and cookies.

There aren't any evidence-based studies on this diet yet, but the anecdotal evidence from the top SIBO researchers in the US suggests that it's worth considering. For more information, including detailed food lists, check out www.goodlfe.com.

Other Carbohydrate-Modified Diet Experiments

There are a handful of other diets designed to remove carbohydrate foods that may increase bloating, abdominal pain, gas, and other IBS symptoms. None of these diets have as much data to support them as the low FODMAP diet, but you may find that the unique, customized approach to carb eating they encourage may address your unique IBS causes. So if you got some relief from the low FODMAP diet but still have some symptoms, you could consider Iterative Action Experiments with these diets to see if they address your unique causes.

SPECIFIC CARBOHYDRATE DIET EXPERIMENT

Initially developed in 1951 as a diet to treat celiac patients, the Specific Carbohydrate Diet (SCD) removes specific types of complex carbohydrates that are harder to digest. This includes:

- All processed sugars
- A majority of grains like corn, wheat, oats, and rice
- Starchy vegetables like potatoes and carrots

SCD is a very restrictive diet template and should only be considered after less limiting diet options haven't helped your gut. For more support with the SCD diet, check out www.scd-forlife.com or consult with a coach, dietitian, or nutritionist.

FAST TRACT DIET EXPERIMENT

Dr. Norm Robillard developed the Fast Tract Diet specifically for his patients with IBS, SIBO, and other reflux and digestive issues.

This diet limits many of the same foods as the low

FODMAP and SDC diets but also eliminates resistant starches, which, according to Dr. Robillard, have fermentation potential. Here is a list of hard-to-digest carbohydrates that Dr. Robillard suggests should be avoided on this diet.

Category	Foods
Resistant starch	Rice, potatoes, grains, and pasta.
Lactose	All dairy products, including milk, cream, ice cream, butter, cheese, etc.
Fructose	Polymeric forms: bananas, apples, grapes, and oranges.
Fiber	Fiber supplements (like Metamucil), whole grains, legumes, and bran.
Sugar alcohols	Foods sweetened with sugar alcohols such as xylitol, erythritol, mannitol, etc.

Table 7: Foods to avoid on the Fast Tract Diet.

This diet uses a fermentation point (FP) system for each food you eat. You keep track of this with the *Fast Tract* app which allows you to check, journal, and track your progress.

So again, if you got partial results from the low FODMAP diet but want to see if you can take it further, you could test this dietary theory with an Iterative Action Experiment and see what your body has to say about it. For more information, visit www.fasttractdiet.com.

Other Possible IBS Food Mediators

Not all IBS food-related symptoms are caused by fermentable carbohydrates. If you have done one of the preceding carbohydrate-reducing diet experiments and saw no symptom relief, chances are a different mediator is causing your IBS food symptoms. Here are a few other options that may be helpful to experiment with if you didn't find relief from these other diets.

· · ·

Low Histamine Diet Experiment

If you've ever taken antihistamine medication, you may be aware that histamine is connected to allergy symptoms.

Histamine is a neurotransmitter that can affect the brain, spinal cord, and gut. Your cells may release histamine when they're exposed to allergens you're sensitive to. Histamine release causes symptoms such as itching, swelling, hives, watery eyes, runny nose, or flushing. Histamine release can also cause digestive symptoms, like diarrhea, nausea, vomiting, or abdominal pain.

Histamine also naturally occurs in some foods and drinks, such as aged meats, alcoholic beverages, and chocolate.

If you react to high-histamine foods or drinks, this is called histamine intolerance, and it can often be an underlying mechanism of IBS symptoms.

Are you sensitive to histamine foods? Here is a list.

Vegetables & Fruits	Meats, Nuts & Dairy	Grains & Other
Fermented vegetables (sauerkraut, pickles, relishes, and olives in vinegar) Avocado Eggplant Spinach Mushrooms Pumpkin Apricots Cherries Bananas Cranberries Citrus fruit Pineapple Raspberries Dates Kiwi Mango Strawberries Dried fruit	Meat (aged, smoked, processed and leftover meat that hasn't been frozen) Fish and shellfish (unless immediately fresh) Fermented soy (tofu, miso, tempeh) Raw eggs (especially egg whites) Long-cooked bone broth Peanuts Cashews Sunflower seeds Walnuts Fermented dairy (blue cheese, yogurt, kefir, buttermilk, etc)	Buckwheat Wheat Soybeans Red beans Alcohol (especially red wine) Kombucha Cinnamon Curry powder Chili powder Paprika Cloves Nutmeg Vinegar and vinegar dressings Soy sauce Yeast Sometimes chocolate

Table 8: Partial high histamine food list.

If many of these foods are on your list of things that worsen your symptoms, it may be worthwhile to do an Iterative Action Experiment with the Low Histamine Diet.

Eating a zero histamine diet is impossible, so your goal is to reduce your histamine intake for two to three weeks and see if your symptoms improve. If so, this strongly suggests histamine is a significant mechanism (or cause) of your IBS symptoms. If not, you'll need to test a different mediator.

SIBO BI-PHASIC DIET EXPERIMENT

If you found partial relief from either the low FODMAP or low histamine diet but still feel like you're reacting to foods, the Bi-Phasic Diet may be helpful. This diet, developed by Dr. Nirala Jacobi and Dr. Heidi Turner, reduces *both* FODMAPs and high histamine foods.

The diet is called "bi-phasic" because it has two phases:

- **Phase 1:** You avoid fermentable, high histamine, and histamine-liberating (foods that can trigger the release of histamine) foods for 2-4 weeks.
- **Phase 2:** You do careful, staged reintroductions to map and understand which of these foods are your symptom triggers.

Though the Bi-Phasic diet is very restrictive and can be challenging to follow, I have had a handful of clients for whom it was very helpful. For more information about the SIBO Bi-Phasic Diet, visit www.sibodoctor.com.

LOW OXALATE DIET EXPERIMENT

Oxalates are naturally occurring substances that are found

in all living beings. People with a healthy digestive system can digest and excrete oxalates just fine. But in some people with IBS and other gut problems, oxalates can be irritating and contribute to symptoms.

I made this connection when I realized that some of my worst gut pain offenders were high oxalate foods like chia, chocolate, and almonds.

People who are sensitive to oxalates primarily experience pain symptoms, but can also have headaches, abdominal or stomach pain, eye pain, diarrhea, and bloating.

So if you experience a lot of joint pain, gut pain, or headaches, and your normal diet contains a lot of high-oxalate foods, it might be worth doing an Iterative Action Experiment to see whether oxalates are one of your food-symptom mediators.

There is also a connection between fungus and oxalates because fungus produces oxalates. So if you've been diagnosed with a fungal overgrowth like *Candida*, and several high-oxalate foods made it to your negative mediator list in your assessment, you might consider trying to reduce oxalates to see if this improves things.

The highest oxalate foods include:

Fruits and Veggies	Nuts, Seeds, and Misc	Grains and Legumes
Spinach and chard Kale Sweet potatoes and yams Beets Rhubarb Celery Green beans Russet potatoes Guava Plantain	Almonds Peanuts Sesame Seeds Chia seeds Many nuts	Wheat (gluten) Buckwheat Amaranth Quinoa Soybeans Many legumes

Table 9: Common high oxalate foods.

IMPORTANT: Doing a low-oxalate diet is different from doing other elimination diets. If you suddenly reduce your oxalate intake, your body can release stores of oxalates. This can suddenly make your symptoms a lot worse. **To safely do a low-oxalate diet, it's necessary to gradually reduce your daily oxalate intake over a week to 10 days.**

As with FODMAPs and histamines, it's impossible to eat a zero-oxalate diet, so the goal with this therapeutic diet is to bring your daily oxalates down to a maximum of 40-60 mg per day. The Trying Low Oxalates Facebook group is the most comprehensive resource about dietary oxalates. The host, Sally Oh, maintains extensive lists of foods and their oxalate content.

As with other therapeutic diets, you'll reduce your oxalate intake for a few weeks and evaluate whether or not you feel better. If not, oxalates are not an issue for you. You can move on to testing a different hypothesis.

If you do feel better, move on to reintroductions to discover which particular high-oxalate foods are your worst triggers.

Paleo Diet Experiment

The Paleo diet has been very popular in integrative health circles for about the last ten years, and with good reason. Many people who switch to a Paleo diet lose weight, have more energy, and see other benefits to their overall health.

Eating a Paleo diet means eating foods our human ancestors would have eaten. This means that you avoid anything processed or foods that came into human civilization after the Agricultural Revolution.

This includes:

- Grains and legumes
- Refined sugars

- Processed foods
- Dairy products
- Refined vegetable oils

The Paleo diet will not necessarily benefit your IBS, and there aren't any studies that recommend it for the syndrome, but it may help if your symptoms are being driven by grains, legumes, sugars, and dairy products. You'll notice that these foods are closely related to the high FODMAP food list.

I find that the Paleo diet is most likely to help if you are currently eating a very mainstream diet full of wheat, dairy, grains, and sweets. If this is where you're starting with your diet, the Paleo diet may be a reasonable dietary Iterative Action Experiment to begin with.

A word of caution about the Paleo diet: Many Paleo recipes substitute nut-based flours for grain flours, so that you can enjoy delicious treats. However, nut flours are super high in FODMAPs. Paleo recipes also often rely on chia seeds, spinach, almonds, sweet potatoes, and chocolate, which are high-oxalate foods. So if you switch to a Paleo diet and feel worse, you might evaluate your sensitivity to oxalates.

The *Whole 30* comprehensive 30-day Paleo elimination diet by Melissa Urban is a great starting point for those interested in experimenting with this diet. The recipes are easy to prepare and super delicious, showing that even if you remove some foods from your life, you can still enjoy eating.

NO MATTER WHICH DIET YOU TEST OUT, BE SURE TO APPROACH IT with a solid question you're trying to answer and observe your body's response carefully. If you see positive results, then you've discovered one of your symptom mechanisms and you can use this information to create an effective symptom management plan. If you don't see any changes or things get worse, this is a sign that you're barking up the wrong tree and need to look elsewhere to find your symptom mechanisms.

Therapeutic Diets Less Likely to Work for IBS

There are many other possible dietary theories, and you may wonder if they would be helpful for you. I'll discuss a few diets that I have generally found don't usually address IBS mechanisms or can be harmful if used inappropriately.

Although the diets I'm about to share may be useful options for some people in some situations, for the most part, you'll find that these diets may aggravate and complicate your IBS healing journey.

Keto Diet

The ketogenic (keto) diet is all the rage right now, and with good reason. As a very low carbohydrate, moderate protein, and high-fat diet, the keto diet can help people lose weight, improve their metabolic health, heal diabetes, and improve Multiple Sclerosis (MS) and Alzheimer's disease. A significant percentage of Americans struggle with these very health concerns. However, there's no research to support its use in IBS. And anecdotally, I've seen the keto diet significantly worsen IBS patients' symptoms.

The reason for this comes down to the mechanisms of the diet. The keto diet has a relatively high proportion of fats. Some people with IBS have a hard time digesting fats, so a high-fat diet could really increase diarrhea and other symptoms. The very low level of carbohydrates can also reduce beneficial bacteria populations in your gut microbiome because they feed on your dietary carbs and fiber. Some versions of the keto diet may also increase your vegetable intake, which might lead to too much fiber, and, therefore more IBS symptoms, especially if you increase high FODMAP veggies.

I personally know the dangers of using the keto diet at the wrong moment. The keto diet was the first therapeutic diet I tried on my IBS journey, and though I appreciate how it helped me break my sugar addiction, the increase in fats and proteins worsened my digestive symptoms. And because I didn't have a strategy for experimenting with diets yet, I doggedly stuck with the diet longer than I should have.

This is why it is so vitally important for you to use the Iterative Action Model to guide your diet change. It's also vitally important to pay attention to how the diet change affects your body. If you don't, you can make your situation far worse.

AUTOIMMUNE PALEO DIET AND LOW-LECTIN DIET

The Autoimmune Paleo diet (AIP) is a more specific Paleo diet that removes foods that may aggravate autoimmune diseases, such as Hashimoto's thyroiditis, Sjögren's disease, and Inflammatory Bowel Disease (IBD).

Like the Paleo diet, this diet avoids sugars, grains, and legumes but also omits eggs, seeds, nuts, nightshades, and seed-sourced spices before completing reintroductions to determine which foods are triggering symptoms.

The Low-Lectin Diet, developed by Dr. Gundry, has a similar approach, but I believe it attempts to address a similar symptom mechanism (immune reactivity to plant compounds).

There is no evidence to suggest that either the Autoimmune Paleo diet or the low-lectin diet would be useful for IBS and other gut conditions, so they're not my go-to options for my clients. That said, you can always decide to do an Iterative

Action Experiment and decide for yourself if your body responds well to the diet.

Because these two diets are quite restrictive, it's essential to work toward reintroductions as soon as possible to avoid malnutrition.

CARNIVORE DIET

As the name states, the carnivore diet removes everything that is not pure protein or animal fat (including some dairy).

Certain people find that this diet relieves gut symptoms thanks to the complete removal of fiber-rich foods like vegetables, nuts, and fruits.

The carnivore diet is often an option of last resort for people with severely reactive guts. However, I feel strongly that the carnivore diet is not a viable long-term diet strategy.

If you cannot eat anything but animal products, this is a strong signal that there may be something much bigger than simply IBS going on. Thinking functionally, this suggests there may be an immune system or autoimmune problem. If you're in this boat, I suggest working with a skilled practitioner to investigate possible deeper underlying causes.

VEGAN/VEGETARIAN/PLANT-BASED DIET

I might take some heat for this, but I don't typically see people with IBS getting better from vegan or vegetarian diets. There are exceptions to this rule, and if you're one of those people who healed your gut with a plant-based diet, I'm happy for you.

More often what I see is IBS patients thinking that this will solve their problem but then finding they feel worse. If you've read this chapter up to this point, you'll know that the likely reason is due to the high levels of fermentable carbohydrates in plant-based diets.

Vegetarians and vegans rely on non-animal sources of protein, including whole grains and legumes, such as brown rice and beans, as well as fermented foods like tofu and tempeh, nuts, and seed or legume-based protein powders. The challenge for people experiencing IBS is that beans, whole grains, ferments, nuts, pea protein powder, and the like are all common IBS symptom triggers. This diet also increases your reliance on veggies and fruits, many of which are also IBS symptom triggers.

I don't dispute that plant-based foods are healthy for the body and the planet! The problem is that many of these foods are common triggers for IBS symptoms.

If you wish to eat a plant-based diet and tame your IBS, I encourage you to do your due diligence with discovering your food-symptom triggers and mediators, and *then* work to create a vegetarian or vegan nutrition plan that works around those sensitivities. The one exception to this is if your food-symptoms are being triggered by difficulty digesting animal protein. In this case, removing meat from your diet could be a worthwhile Iterative Action Experiment to assess how you feel.

What If You Don't Know Which Diet to Start With?

Selecting a diet option is easier if you already have some sense of which foods are causing you trouble. But what if you really don't know which foods are bothering you? I periodically hear from people who are very confused about this.

There are two main approaches you can take to try and get some clarity about this.

One is to do a series of elimination diets, like I've discussed in this chapter, to try and figure out your food-symptom mechanism. I generally recommend a staged elimination process that starts at the general and works toward the more specific.

So, for example, if you haven't yet made any changes to your diet, start with a simple elimination diet, like the Paleo diet, that removes the top four most common problem foods: gluten, dairy, sugar, and alcohol.

If that doesn't help, or helps a little but not all the way, then you can choose a more restrictive option and see if you can get more clarity about the mechanism behind your food-related symptoms. So for our example, perhaps then you would then try the low FODMAP or low histamine diet.

But sometimes, no matter how diligent you are with your food-based Iterative Action Experiments, you still don't know what's triggering your problem. This is where some old-fashioned sleuthing comes in.

Find Your Mystery Food-Symptom Triggers With Tracking

If none of the above food eliminations work, then I recommend a specific type of food-symptom tracking called a Food, Mood, Poop (FMP) journal. This technique was taught to me by my mentor and teacher Andrea Nakayama at the Functional Nutrition Alliance.

Food, Mood, Poop tracking is a way to learn from your actual observations of your body. For a few days, commit to tracking what you ate and when, your signs and symptoms, and what kind of bowel movements you had and when.

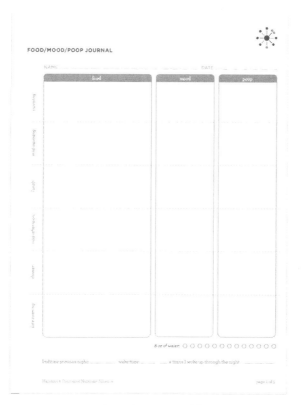

Figure 3: Food, Mood, Poop Journal from Andrea Nakayama and the Functional Nutrition Alliance. Used with permission.

Believe it or not, studying your bowel movements can give you important information about how your gut tolerates the food you eat. For consistency, you'll use the Bristol Stool Chart, a standardized pictorial guide to poop, to determine which type of poop you had.

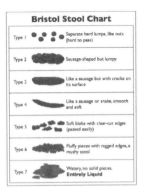

Figure 4: Bristol stool chart.

FMP tracking should continue for at least five days, but it may take more days of tracking to find enough data to work with. Once you've collected that data, you'll look for times when you were experiencing symptoms you'd like to have less of. It's best to find at least two to three incidences and compare them.

Then you can ask yourself, what was similar between them? Are there any foods in common? If you see something that looks like it may be a culprit, you can now design an Iterative Action Experiment to test your theory.

I used this method to figure out that broccoli was triggering my constipation one to two days after eating it. I had three weeks or so of data, and I went through my log with a highlighter and found all the incidences of constipation. What I would never have figured out without the FMP journal was that every time I skipped a day of pooping, I had eaten broccoli one to two days before.

So I tested the hypothesis by eating broccoli and tracking my symptoms and poop on my FMP journal. Once again, I skipped a day of pooping. *Bingo!*

No matter how weird or confusing your food symptoms get, you can use this method to figure out what might be triggering your food reactions and create an Iterative Action Experiment to test your theory.

Should You Use a Food Sensitivity Test to Find Your IBS Food Triggers?

My clients and subscribers often ask if food sensitivity tests can help detect IBS triggers.

Common food sensitivity tests such as the ALCAT, CYREX panels, Mediator Release Test (MRT), and Everlywell test a sample of your blood to look for an IgG immune reaction to a collection of foods. Your test result typically includes color-coded graphs showing which foods were reactive.

I don't generally recommend IgG food sensitivity tests for several reasons.

The biggest reason is that these tests only look for *one type* of reaction to foods. I hope you understand from reading this chapter that there are many possible reasons for IBS food reactions. *This test only looks for one possibility: an IgG immune reaction.* Reactions to FODMAP or high histamine foods do not register on these tests, and these are far more likely to be the cause of your IBS symptoms.

Some evidence suggests that an IgG response is simply an indicator of what you've previously been exposed to or eaten and may not even signify a problem.

Usually, these test results confuse my clients and make them more anxious about what they need to do. A far better approach is to consider what you think is the mechanism of your food symptoms and to do your own Iterative Action Experiments to test that theory. You'll get much higher-quality answers.

The one time when I do recommend food sensitivity tests is when a thorough series of diet experiments doesn't reveal which foods are causing a problem. At this stage, the IgG test would be a reasonable Iterative Action Experiment, followed by an elimination diet and reintroductions to test the validity of the results you got on the test.

Tips for Success With Dietary Iterative Action Experiments

Many of my clients feel overwhelmed and anxious about changing their diets or are simply exhausted with having to think so much about what they should or shouldn't eat. I certainly had moments in my journey where I felt this way too. Can you relate?

Here's how to make diet changes without overwhelm.

TIP 1: FOOD CHANGES DON'T NEED TO BE ALL-OR-NOTHING. IT *IS* true that making big changes may help you get to your goal faster, but if doing so overwhelms you to the point where you can't do it, this will certainly lead to failure! Feel free to slow down the process of food eliminations by focusing on one or a few foods at a time. In other words, structure your experiment to set yourself up for success.

TIP 2: PREPARE FOR YOUR EXPERIMENT BEFORE STARTING. Whether you'll be starting with small or grand changes, prepare for your experiment by shopping appropriately. Work with food lists, sample meal plans, or recipes to think about what you'll be eating and how to adapt your normal diet. Make sure you have compliant foods on hand so you don't get caught feeling hungry with nothing to eat!

. . .

Tip 3: Keep it simple. Sometimes, when people try out a new diet, they want to try complicated new recipes. It usually works better for my clients when they try to maintain their normal menu, but with a few tweaks or swaps. For example, if you're removing gluten, you can still eat pasta, just swap out gluten-free pasta for a wheat one. Or, if you're trying new things, I encourage you to find simple, easy recipes and stick to those.

Tip 4: Get your family members' support. Changing your diet can bring up a lot of feelings: anxiety, fear, anger, or frustration. It can also be challenging for your family. If you can, explain to your family why you're making these changes and see if they're willing to go on the journey with you to show support. If they don't want to, maybe your partner is willing to take over family food prep so you can focus on your experiment. Doing hard things is easier if our loved ones are backing us up.

Tip 5: Don't dwell in food purgatory forever. Do your best to determine your food-symptom mechanisms with the methods explained in this chapter. But if you aren't getting anywhere after a few months, moving on to other things is okay. (See Chapters 5, 6, and 7) In this case, food may not be a significant part of your problem. Also, don't stay on the elimination phase of *any* diet for more than a month before moving on to reintroductions.

5

SUPPORT YOUR BASIC DIGESTIVE FUNCTION

Though we eat almost every day of our lives, few of us think very much about how our digestion works. It's supposed to do its job in the background without much fuss. It's supposed to digest your food, absorb it, and send those nutrients wherever they need to go to power everything you do, from sleeping or exercising to thinking and breathing.

But if you're reading this book, chances are your digestive system is in some state of rebellion. It's not doing what it should be. The good news is that you can support your most foundational digestive functions with some simple Iterative Action Experiments. In some cases, these basic supports can profoundly influence how well you digest and absorb your food.

Let's begin with a tour of your digestive system and talk about how things should work. I'd like to educate you about your digestive anatomy and processes because it's helpful to understand which parts may not be working right. It's also helpful to understand where the parts are located so that you can best estimate which organ is hurting or not feeling right.

This can be helpful as you assess what you need support with or during a conversation with your doctor.

Digestion 101

Your digestive system is beautifully designed to transform the food you eat into cell power. It's the first organ system, besides the heart, to form in a developing baby. You use it every single day when you eat your meals and drink beverages. But though each of us has one, many have no idea how it works or where to find the various organs.

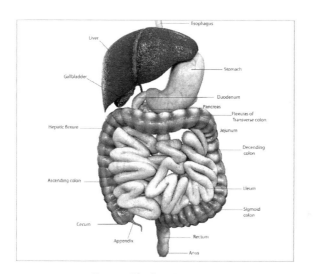

Figure 4: The digestive system.

THE BRAIN & NERVOUS SYSTEM

It may not seem like the brain is a part of your digestive system, but it plays a significant role in your digestion. Before you even sit down to eat, you begin thinking about, smelling, or looking at food. This not only triggers your hunger but it stimulates the release of your digestive juices. Your nervous system also controls all the involuntary movements required to send your food through your body, everything from swallowing to pooping. However, stress can derail this cascade of events, and significantly impact your digestive function. This is why stress relief practices can be so powerful at resetting your digestion.

The Mouth, Salivary Glands, and Chewing

Your mouth and salivary glands are the first physical part of your digestive system. Though we don't often think of it this way, physical digestion begins in your mouth with chewing. As you chew your food, your salivary glands secrete saliva, and your tongue and teeth mash up your food to mix it with your saliva. This first stage of digestion is both mechanical and chemical. Saliva particularly helps digest carbohydrates. As we discussed in Chapter 2, the longer you spend chewing, the easier time the rest of your digestive system has to do its job.

The Esophagus

Your esophagus is the tube that runs from your mouth to your stomach. It passes behind your heart, which is why you can experience pain in your heart area when you have acid reflux (also known as heartburn). After chewing your food, you swallow the bite of food and it passes through your esophagus with an involuntary wave-like motion called peristalsis, and enters your stomach.

The Stomach

Your stomach is located on the left side of your abdomen, under and below the rib cage. The stomach secretes hydrochloric acid and mechanically churns your chewed-up food to further mix it with your digestive juices. The resulting material is called chyme, and your stomach slowly releases it, bit by bit, into the small intestine.

Stomach acid provides many important functions for your digestion. It helps break proteins down into their most basic building blocks (amino acids and peptides) for absorption, and protects you from incoming pathogens, like bacteria or parasites. It's part of the trigger mechanism for your body to secrete pancreatic enzymes and bile from your gallbladder. It also helps you absorb vitamin B12, iron, and zinc.

THE SMALL INTESTINE (SMALL BOWEL), PANCREAS, LIVER, AND Gallbladder

The small intestine is the star of the nutrient absorption show. Your small intestine has three parts: the duodenum, jejunum, and ileum. It's located roughly between your belly button and your pubic bone.

As the chyme enters your small intestine, it triggers the release of pancreatic enzymes and bile from your gallbladder. The enzymes (amylase, lipase, and protease) further break down the carbohydrates, fats, and proteins and help transport them across the lining of your small intestine. Bile, which is made in your liver and is stored in your gallbladder, helps emulsify your fats so they can be better absorbed.

Tiny, finger-like projections called "villi," which make the inside of your small intestine look like a shag carpet, line the small intestine. If you were to flatten the inside of your small intestine, it would have the area of a tennis court! Each of these villi absorbs specific nutrients. The villi are only one cell thick.

Between meals, your autonomic nervous system (rest-and-digest state) initiates cleaning waves in your small intestine to completely move things through. These cleaning waves begin 2-3 hours after you last ate, and the strongest waves happen during your long overnight fast. Weak or non-existent cleaning waves are thought to be one of the main reasons SIBO develops (Pimentel, et. al., 2002). This is why it's important to minimize snacking if you have SIBO.

Your liver is located up under and partly below your rib cage on your right side, and your gallbladder is a small sac underneath your liver. The liver is one of your two main detoxification organs (your kidneys are the other). Using complex biochemical processes, it breaks down hormones, chemicals, alcohol, and more into more benign compounds so they can be excreted in your stool.

THE LARGE INTESTINE (LARGE BOWEL)

Your large intestine provides the final stage of digestion, where the last bit of absorption occurs. The large bowel starts in your lower right abdomen at the ileocecal valve, travels up almost to your rib cage, drapes across your abdomen at about the level of your belly button, and then drops down your left side toward your rectum.

Your large bowel is where liquids and minerals are absorbed, and this is also where your beneficial bacteria live. These bacteria provide you with vitamins, short-chain fatty acids, and fermentation by-products.

Once the waste material reaches your rectum, it's stored until your digestive system signals that it's time to eliminate. If things are working normally, a complex, coordinated relay of neurological and physical actions signals your anus to release a bowel movement, and the digestive process is complete.

Iterative Action Experiments to Support Your Natural Digestive Function

In reading through this previous section, did you learn new things about your digestive system? Did anything stand out to you as something your gut may need help with?

You may have begun to get a sense of which organs may need some help. The good news is we can support and enhance your normal and natural digestive function in several ways.

In many cases, the simple supports I'm going to share with you can provide surprising relief. And even if it only makes a small difference, I find that supporting your gut at this level prepares your body to handle any future, deeper-level treatments you may need.

There are three main digestive support Iterative Action Experiments worth testing to see how your gut responds: probiotics, stomach acid support, and digestive enzymes. Let's explore how to do experiments with these options.

Using Probiotics as an Iterative Action Experiment

Probiotics are beneficial bacteria that naturally and normally live in your gut, on your skin, and all your mucous membranes. You can find up to approximately 500 species in your gut at any time.

In some ways, our understanding of probiotics is still in its infancy; but every year, we learn more about the wide range of benefits they provide us with. Research has shown that probiotics:

- Decrease gut inflammation (Hedin et. al., 2007; Kruis et. al., 2004)

- Can help treat pathogenic gut infections (Eslami et. al., 2014; Besirbellioglu et. al., 2006)
- Improve IBS symptoms, including bloating and abdominal pain, and in some cases, diarrhea or constipation (Yuan et. al., 2017; Tiequn et. al., 2015; Wheelan, 2011; Ford et. al., 2014).
- Can improve leaky gut (Lamprecht et. al., 2012)
- Can improve non-digestive symptoms, such as skin conditions (Muizzuddin, 2012), depression (Ng et. al., 2018), vaginal infections (Wang et. al., 2019), and more.

Given all these benefits and the ample research showing their benefits for gut conditions, it's reasonable for you to try an Iterative Action Experiment with probiotics to see if your gut can benefit.

However, it's important to approach this experiment with the right strategy. The first thing you might be wondering about is which types of probiotics you should use.

Though there are hundreds, if not thousands, of probiotic products on the market, according to Doctor of Naturopathic Medicine Michael Ruscio, there are generally three common types of probiotics: *Lactobacillus* and *Bifidobacteria* blends, *Saccharomyces boulardii* (a beneficial yeast), and soil-based probiotics. Most people who try probiotics use a *Lactobacillus* and *Bifidobacteria* blend. If they find it doesn't help, they give up on it.

Research suggests that using diverse probiotic strains provides better results than only using one type (Zhang et. al., 2020). So a full trial of probiotics is best done by trying all three types together to increase your bacterial diversity, as long as you can tolerate them.

Dr. Ruscio uses this strategy in his clinic with his patients and receives generally positive results. So rather than trying each of the hundreds of probiotics products, you simply need to find one high-quality product per category and trial that with the Iterative Action Method.

Many people ask me which specific probiotic products they should use, and there is no one right answer for everyone. Here is a list of criteria to help you choose quality probiotics. Look for products that:

- List the specific species or strains of bacteria.
- Show the potency, or colony-forming units, in the billions.
- Do not contain allergens like gluten or dairy. Some commercial products gastroenterologists recommend contain dairy-derived ingredients, which may be problematic for dairy-sensitive IBS patients. Double-check the ingredients if you're not sure.
- Is refrigerated (unless they're soil-based probiotics, which are usually shelf stable).

Here is a list of brands I recommend to clients that generally meet these requirements. This is not an exhaustive or complete list.

- Seeking Health
- Microbiome Labs
- KLAIRE Labs
- Pure Encapsulations
- Allergy Research Group
- Dr. Ruscio's Functional Medicine Formulations

Tips for Using Probiotics as an Iterative Action Experiment

Tip 1: Only start one new thing at a time. Though I'm recommending trying three types of probiotics, I highly recommend only starting one new product at a time. This way, if you react badly, you'll know which one is responsible.

TIP 2: START LOW AND GO SLOW. YOUR BODY MAY NOT NEED THE full, recommended therapeutic dose. Especially for people with sensitive tummies, I suggest starting with less than the full dose and slowly working up to the recommended amount. So, for example, if the label recommends two capsules twice a day, start with one capsule once per day for a few days, or even a half capsule, and assess how you feel. If all is well, you can add another and slowly work up to your best therapeutic dose.

TIP 3: CHECK FOR PREBIOTIC INGREDIENTS IN YOUR PROBIOTICS. Many probiotics include prebiotic fiber as a food source for the bacteria. But if you're sensitive to FODMAPs, these ingredients may increase your bloating, gas, or abdominal pain. If you've reacted to probiotics previously, this may be the reason. Read the product labels carefully, and if you're sensitive to FODMAPs, avoid ingredients such as inulin, galacto-oligosaccharides (GOS), fructo-oligosaccharides (FOS), and so on.

TIP 4: USE PROBIOTICS WHEN THEY'RE CONVENIENT FOR YOU. Many sources recommend using probiotics on an empty stomach, at bedtime, or with meals. Which one is right? Ideally, on an empty stomach is preferable; but if this isn't possible for some reason, it's okay to use them whenever they work for you.

. . .

Tip 5: If you have confirmed or suspected SIBO, it may be best to avoid probiotics for now. There is conflicting research about whether or not probiotics are helpful for SIBO. A meta-analysis suggests that they are helpful (Zhong et. al., 2017), while Dr. Pimentel, the leading SIBO researcher in the US, says he generally recommends against them because he often sees them flare his patients. The truth is probably somewhere in between. You'll have to decide for yourself whether to try this or not, and to see how your body responds.

Stomach Acid Support as an Iterative Action Experiment

As I mentioned earlier, stomach acid provides several very important functions for your digestion. It not only helps with protein digestion, but also stimulates the secretion of your bile and enzymes, and helps with absorption of iron, zinc, and vitamin B12.

There are several situations where an Iterative Action Experiment of stomach acid support would be indicated:

- If you've noticed that you don't seem to digest proteins well.
- Your digestion seems to move very slowly.
- You frequently get stomach bugs or food poisoning.
- Your iron, zinc, or B12 levels are low on blood tests.
- Reflux or heartburn can indicate too much or too little stomach acid.

Here are two simple ways to increase stomach acid production:

Add lemon juice or apple cider vinegar to your diet	Drink about ½-1 tbsp of lemon juice or apple cider vinegar in a few ounces of water just before your meal.
Add betaine hydrochloric acid capsules to your daily routine.	Take one capsule of betaine HCL before your meals. You can increase up to 2-3 caps per meal, but more than that shouldn't be necessary.

Table 10: Ways to support stomach acid.

Choose one of these options and use them for a few weeks, and then ask yourself if any of your symptoms have changed. If so, you've found one of your underlying symptom mechanisms. If not, move on to testing other options.

Don't use stomach acid supplementation if:

- You have or suspect an active *H. pylori* infection.
- You have or suspect SIBO, as recent research suggests it may feed the bacteria that produce hydrogen (Wietesman et. al., 2022).
- Have active stomach ulcers.

Also, use it with caution if you have heartburn or reflux. For some people, it clears it up quickly. For others, it makes it worse. If stomach acid support worsens your reflux, this is a strong message from your body to stop.

Incorporating Digestive Enzymes, Bitters, & Bile as an Iterative Action Experiment

Your pancreas produces and releases enzymes to help you digest your food as your gut moves food through your system. Sometimes, your pancreas doesn't produce enough enzymes to do the job effectively.

This is called "Exocrine Pancreatic Insufficiency" (EPI) in severe cases. This condition is the cause of IBS in only a small percentage of cases, so it's less likely to be your primary underlying cause. That said, your body can be just a little deficient in enzymes, and digestive enzyme supplements may improve your digestive function.

If you feel like your digestion could use a little support, you can do an Iterative Action Experiment with digestive enzyme capsules or tablets by taking them just before your meals. **Look for enzyme products that contain pancreatin, which includes amylase, lipase, and protease.** You can also experiment with enzyme supplements that support the digestion of other foods, like lactase to help with lactose or cellulase to help with cellulose. As with most experiments, test them for two to three weeks and assess whether your digestive symptoms have improved.

For some people, digestive enzymes can increase gut irritation. If this happens, this is a clear message from your body that enzymes are not for you at this time.

Another way to support your natural digestive enzyme production is to use digestive bitters before your meal or incorporate bitter foods into your meals. The bitterness will activate excess saliva (thus enzyme secretion) in your mouth and the rest of your gut to help with digestion.

One additional support supplement that can help with fat digestion is bile salts. As I mentioned on our tour of the digestive system, bile is produced in your liver and stored in your gallbladder.

If your gallbladder was removed, you may have less capacity to tolerate a high-fat meal. Supplementing with bile salts (ox bile or TUDCA) may be helpful to improve your fat digestion. You can do an Iterative Action Experiment with this to see whether it improves your symptoms.

In Summary

A wide variety of supplements can be used to help improve your baseline digestive function. But it's important to understand that you probably won't need to use *all* of these options. The point of using the Iterative Action process is to find which specific ones really benefit you, and to only use those things which are truly helpful.

As with the majority of the treatments I discuss in this book, the goal isn't to stay on these supports forever, but only as long as they're helpful and they bring about a beneficial change.

Approach your experiments with a good question and hypothesis, and see what you can learn about your underlying symptom mechanisms from those experiments. If there is no improvement, then you put them aside and move on to the next step.

6

WHAT'S THE ROOT CAUSE OF YOUR IBS?

At the beginning of this book, I said that this is the million-dollar question for IBS patients everywhere. Many patients are looking for the one single answer to this question, hoping that if they find it, they can fix it. But because IBS is a syndrome, there often isn't one clear answer to this question.

There are likely to be several overlapping causes that need attention. It's rare, in my experience, that there is one single underlying cause that resolves IBS. Alzheimer's researcher Dr. Dale Bredesen often says that addressing the root causes of Alzheimer's is like needing to plug 36 holes in the roof. I think of IBS in a similar way. You need to consider all the different contributors to the problem and address as many as you can.

However, I hope that in reading up to this point, you can see that the answers you'll get from your Iterative Action Experiments can reveal some of your root causes.

For example, if you found that managing your stress with meditation helps, then stress is part of your root causes. If you found that high-histamine foods worsen your symptoms, then histamine intolerance is one of your root causes. And if you found that betaine HCL dramatically improved your symptoms, then low stomach acid is one of your root causes. These are all valid and true root causes, and addressing each appropriately helps you find your path to symptom resolution.

But what's causing *those* problems? Sometimes, these problems are branches off of a larger trunk. Now that you've done everything you can to manage your symptoms, it's time to look deeper and explore what might be lying beneath.

So in this chapter, I'll discuss some of the deeper known true root causes of IBS and how you can begin investigating whether they are *your* root causes.

While there's no way to list all the possible IBS root causes, there are patterns. A relatively short list causes the vast majority. Most of these root causes will require investigation with a medical doctor, Naturopath, or Health Coach, but it's helpful to have some idea of where to start. Let's explore what may be at the most root level of your IBS.

Gut Infections as IBS Root Causes

One of the most commonly overlooked root causes of IBS are gut infections. Doctors do generally widely accept that previous infections can lead to the syndrome, and this concept of "postinfectious IBS" is understood to be a factor for some patients. What doctors often discount is how these infections can linger and continue to affect patients' quality of life far beyond the initial infection. Furthermore, many clinicians in the trenches of general practice don't know how to look for these subclinical infections.

The most common gut infections that may cause IBS include:

- SIBO (Small Intestinal Bacterial Overgrowth)
- Non-SIBO bacterial dysbiosis
- *H. pylori* infection
- *Candida* and other yeasts
- Parasites

One thing that can be kind of confusing is that just because you have a result on a lab test that's positive for an infection, like SIBO for example, doesn't necessarily mean that that infection is what's causing your symptoms. Each test result like this is a hypothesis until proven that it is truly responsible for your symptoms.

For example, if you test positive for SIBO, you won't know if SIBO is truly part of your root causes until you trial a treatment as an Iterative Action Experiment and see how you feel. If you try a round of SIBO treatment and your symptoms improve, this strongly suggests that, yes, SIBO was an underlying cause of your IBS symptoms. If you didn't improve from your treatment, this means you need to look elsewhere for your root cause. And though this can feel disappointing, this is very helpful information to guide your future treatment.

So let's detail some of these common IBS causes and how to confirm whether they are likely affecting you.

SIBO (SMALL INTESTINAL BACTERIAL OVERGROWTH)

According to new research, SIBO (small intestinal bacterial overgrowth) causes approximately 60% of IBS cases. However, SIBO is usually secondary to other causes, so in addition to discovering you have SIBO, you must also ask what's causing your SIBO in the first place.

The most common cause of SIBO is a previous case of food poisoning. The bacteria responsible for the food poisoning releases Cytolethal distending toxin B (CdtB). CdtB affects the signaling of the nerves that control your small intestinal motility. To add insult to injury, CdtB may also make your body begin producing anti-vinculin antibodies, which also attack the mechanism that moves your small intestines. When your small intestine loses its natural motility, this then allows bacteria to overgrow in your small intestine.

But really, anything that impacts your small intestinal motility can lead to SIBO. Other causes of slow small-intestinal motility can include previous abdominal surgeries, like cesarean sections or appendectomies. These events can create adhesions and scar tissue that can affect your motility. A prior car accident or injury could do the same. Medications that slow gut motility (like opioids) could also lead to SIBO.

So it's important to know that even if you find that SIBO is one of your root causes, you need to keep digging to find what caused it in the first place because if you don't address that, your SIBO will continue to recur.

TESTING FOR SIBO

SIBO testing is usually done with a home breath test kit. After eating a 24-hour prep diet, you collect a baseline breath sample. Then, you drink a sugar solution—either lactulose or glucose—and collect breath samples every 15 or 20 minutes, depending on the kit, for 2-3 hours.

I recommend the TrioSmart breath test, which checks for all three known SIBO gasses: hydrogen, methane, and hydrogen sulfide.

If the TrioSmart or other SIBO testing isn't available, I recommend the FoodMarble AIRE 2 device. See the resources section for information about accessing SIBO testing.

. . .

Non-SIBO Dysbiosis

"Dysbiosis" simply means an imbalance of your normal and healthy gut bacteria. If your doctor or naturopath tells you that you have dysbiosis, this doesn't mean you have a specific infection that needs attention. It means that your overall balance of microorganisms needs support.

Though research in this area is still in its infancy, some specific species of bacteria have been shown to cause digestive discomfort if they're overgrown.

Testing for Non-SIBO Dysbiosis

You can test for this type of dysbiosis by using functional stool testing, like the GI MAP (see below) or the Genova GI360 stool test. See the Resources section for information about accessing the GI MAP.

H. Pylori Infection

H. pylori is a pathogenic bacteria that can live anywhere in your digestive tract but tends to live in the stomach. It disrupts the acid-producing cells in the stomach and has been shown to be the primary cause of stomach ulcers.

Many IBS patients who have had a full GI workup, including an endoscopy, have been tested for *H. pylori* by stomach biopsy. However, this method of testing often misses *H. pylori* infection.

It might seem like *H. pylori* shouldn't impact IBS since it lives in the stomach. But if you think about the digestive system as a whole, healthy digestion requires many sequential steps to work well. Remember from our physiology lesson in Chapter 5 that good stomach function is necessary for protein digestion, absorption of certain nutrients, and protection of our gut from pathogens (bad bugs). In this way, if *H. pylori* is present in the most upstream part of your gut, it stands to reason that it can impact your entire digestive system downstream.

A systematic review and meta-analysis study completed by Li and others in 2020 suggests IBS may be more likely in people with an *H. pylori* infection (Li et. al., 2020). My anecdotal evidence supports this view. I've had several clients who were declared *H. pylori*-free by biopsy during endoscopy and found *H. pylori* on DNA-based stool testing. When they treated the infection, their IBS symptoms got dramatically better.

H. pylori likely impacts IBS by destabilizing healthy gut function throughout the digestive system, and it can be a root cause of IBS. I encourage you to consider *H. pylori* as a root cause if you have gastritis, reflux, or heartburn, poor digestive function, slow digestion, or if it feels like your entire digestive system isn't right.

TESTING FOR *H. PYLORI*

There are three ways to test for *H. pylori*:

1. Biopsy during endoscopy
2. Stool test, like the GI MAP
3. Urea Breath test (similar to, but different from, a SIBO breath test).

H. pylori breath testing may be covered by insurance if your doctor determines testing is warranted.

CANDIDA

Candida is a naturally occurring yeast in our digestive system. An overgrowth of Candida can cause IBS-like symptoms. This includes symptoms such as bloating, abdominal pain, and diarrhea, and some of the non-digestive symptoms that go along with IBS, like joint pain, brain fog, headaches, itching and rashes, and so on.

Doctors often overlook Candida as a potential cause of IBS symptoms. This may be because a true Candida overgrowth is a life-threatening systemic infection that mostly affects immuno-compromised people. However, Candida overgrowth can be something to consider as a cause of IBS symptoms, especially if you've frequently used antibiotics in your past, eaten a very high-sugar and high-carb diet, used a lot of alcohol, or have had frequent and recurrent yeast infections.

Candida can be tricky to find in traditional testing, but DNA-PCR stool testing can find candida quite easily and give you a quantitative result, giving you an idea of how severe the overgrowth is.

I encourage you to consider Candida or fungal overgrowth as a root cause if sugar worsens your symptoms or worsens during and after antibiotic treatment.

TESTING FOR CANDIDA

It's difficult to test for Candida. There are no available tests for small intestinal fungal overgrowth (SIFO). But Candida sometimes turns up on stool testing, such as the GI MAP or Genova GI 360. Some functional or naturopathic practitioners will also look for antibodies to Candida in blood testing.

THE ORGANIC ACIDS TEST (OATS), WHICH LOOKS AT VARIOUS metabolites in your urine, can also show indirect evidence of fungal overgrowth. However, there isn't yet clear evidence that this is clinically useful information.

. . .

PARASITES

Parasites are microorganisms like nematodes (worms) or amoebas (protozoa) that can reside in your digestive system and cause havoc. Doctors are typically aware of the possibility of parasites as a cause of digestive distress, especially if you've recently traveled abroad, have swum in freshwater lakes or rivers, or drunk water from wells or springs.

Many people think you can't get parasites while living in developed countries, but this isn't true. Common parasite infections in the US include *Giardia lamblia*, *Cryptosporidium*, *Entamoeba histolytica*, and liver flukes.

Testing for parasites can be tricky because they have complex life cycles with varying stages. A single negative stool test may not be enough to confirm or rule out an infection.

I especially encourage you to consider parasites as a root cause if your symptoms are cyclical or worsen near the full moon. Parasites are more likely to hatch or become more active near the full moon.

TESTING FOR PARASITES

Parasites can be difficult to find, as their activity levels change over time, and some types may even go dormant. For best results, if you suspect you have parasites, test with a DNA-PCR-based stool test like the GI MAP, or use a lab with trained infectious disease experts like the Parasites.org Precise Home Parasite Test Kit (See Resources for how to access). This lab collects two samples a few days apart, and encourages collection near the full moon.

You can also request an "Ova and Parasite" stool testing kit from your regular doctor if your budget prevents you from using a specialty lab.

Non-Infectious Underlying Causes of IBS

Not all underlying causes of IBS are infectious. If you come up empty with testing and evaluation for SIBO and other gut infections, consider one of these other options.

ENDOMETRIOSIS

Endometriosis is a condition where tissue similar to the lining of the uterus (endometrium), exists outside the uterus in the abdominal cavity. These tissues respond to a woman's monthly hormone changes just like the uterus, which means that they swell and then bleed. Internal blood with nowhere to go causes not only excruciating pain but also adhesions. Endometriosis can also cause digestive symptoms akin to IBS, and the ongoing formation of adhesions and scar tissue can lead to SIBO.

According to a 2021 systematic review and meta-analysis, women with endometriosis are at least two times more likely to be diagnosed with IBS than women without (Chiaffarino et. al., 2021). I'm very passionate about raising awareness about the connection between endometriosis and IBS because endometriosis was the true root cause of my digestive symptoms. When my endo would act up, I would have severe bloating, abdominal pain, diarrhea, and cramping.

So if your digestive symptoms flare up with your monthly menstrual periods, and include severe pain, consider investigating endometriosis. Though diagnosing endometriosis can be an invasive process, it's important to have clarity about exactly what is causing your problem so you can find the right treatment path.

TESTING FOR ENDOMETRIOSIS

Unfortunately, there are very limited simple options when it comes to testing for endometriosis. According to endometriosis surgeon and expert Andrew Cook, MD, the best options include:

- Exploratory surgery (laparoscopy) to physically see the endometriosis.
- CA-125 blood level, which is typically a marker for ovarian cancer, but appears to often be elevated in women with endometriosis (Kim et. al., 2019).
- Intravaginal ultrasound done by a skilled and specialized ultrasound tech may be able to visualize endometriomas (large cysts) on the ovaries or adenomyosis (endometriosis in the uterine wall).
- A health history of severely painful periods, heavy menstrual bleeding, and pain with intercourse or bowel movements, as well as IBS symptoms, strongly suggest endometriosis.

Work with your primary doctor or OB/GYN to investigate these options.

STRUCTURAL ISSUES IN YOUR DIGESTIVE SYSTEM

If you have ever been in a serious accident and needed abdominal surgery, or injured yourself in the abdominal region through sporting activities, you may have structural limitations in your digestive system. You can also have altered anatomy that can affect your digestion, such as pelvic floor dysfunction, hernias, or tortuous colon.

Adhesions or scar tissue in your abdomen can impede the normal flow of digestion, and lead to bacterial overgrowth, SIBO, or other problems. Colon prolapse, uterine prolapse, hernias, and other malformations can also prevent normal stool elimination. In extreme cases, this can lead to a bowel obstruction, which is a life-threatening emergency that may require surgery and bowel resection.

Varying kinds of scar tissue develop from previous surgeries, injuries, endometriosis, and chemotherapy. Unfortunately, medical imaging often cannot see these internal structural issues.

Testing for Structural Issues

As with endometriosis, there are limited easy options for assessing structural issues in your digestive system. The following options may help you get some clarity.

- Getting evaluated by a skilled physical therapist or craniosacral therapist with training in visceral massage.
- Evaluation by the Clear Passage clinics (See Resources).
- If you have a history of injury or abdominal surgery, consider structural issues a possible root cause requiring investigation.
- Magnetic Resonance Imaging (MRI) or CT scans may reveal obstructions or other anatomical malformations but may or may not be able to visualize adhesions or scar tissue unless they are quite large.

Autoimmune Disease

Sometimes, despite all manner of investigation and testing, my clients come up empty. If this is the case, and symptoms include swelling, rashes, odd reactions, joint pain, or fatigue, an undiagnosed autoimmune condition may be possible.

Autoimmunity is when your body's immune system misidentifies your own tissues as an invader and begins attacking you. There are hundreds of autoimmune diseases, and many of them can affect your digestive system. One example is Hashimoto's thyroiditis. In this condition, your body attacks your thyroid gland, leading to low thyroid function and levels of thyroid hormone. Low levels of thyroid hormone can cause constipation, among many other symptoms.

So if immune-related symptoms accompany your digestive symptoms, and no diet or lifestyle options have made a difference, consider connecting with a skilled naturopathic physician specializing in autoimmune conditions or a conventional rheumatologist to investigate this as a possible root cause.

Mold Illness

Exposure to mold in your home or workplace can cause problems for some people and their guts.

Many doctors don't recognize the concept that mold can cause illness, but research does suggest that mold exposure can impact the gut lining and microbiome (Liew and Mohd-Redzwan, 2018). If your house or workplace is water damaged, or you suspect you've been exposed to mold, you might consider investigating this as a root cause.

Mold illness is very complicated to investigate, so I recommend working with a mold-literate physician or practitioner who can help you navigate this well. (See Resources for helpful References.)

.   .   .

OTHER ROOT CAUSES

There can be other possible root causes besides the ones I've mentioned here. There are many possibilities.

If you plan to investigate other options, this is fine. Just remember to apply the Iterative Action Method in your investigation. Think about possible mechanisms that could explain your symptoms, create experiments to test your theory, and use what you learn to find answers. Work with qualified practitioners who can help you get to the bottom of things.

Tips for Investigating Your Root Causes

Here are some of my best tips for investigating your possible root causes.

TIP 1: LOOK TO YOUR HEALTH HISTORY FOR CLUES. THINK ABOUT when your symptoms started and ask, "What was happening around the time I got sick?" This exercise often turns up key insights into your initial symptom mechanism and your root cause.

TIP 2: USE WHAT YOU'VE ALREADY LEARNED TO NARROW DOWN **your options.** Use what you already know or can observe about your symptoms and mechanisms to help lead you in the right direction. For example, the onset of my gut symptoms came during a period of very high stress in my life, and the symptoms always got worse with my periods. They also got worse as I entered perimenopause.

It seems obvious now that endometriosis was the cause, but

at the time, it was elusive. The initial onset and hormones as mediators were huge clues that could have led me to a diagnosis and appropriate treatment much sooner.

TIP 3: FIND A DOCTOR OR PRACTITIONER WHO SPECIALIZES IN **your likely problem.** If you think your problem is an undiagnosed autoimmune disease, but you try to get your primary care doctor to help you with that, they won't know what to do (other than offer you a referral). Choosing the right specialist helps you get the right care!

TIP 4: BE **METHODICAL!** ALWAYS START EXPERIMENTING WITH the simplest or most likely causes of your symptoms before testing for or experimenting with the most complex, and keep using what you learn to guide you to your next best steps. I would say that 80% of the time, the reason my incoming clients aren't making meaningful progress with their symptoms is that they're not using a systematic strategy to guide their inquiry.

TIP 5: KEEP TRACK OF YOUR ITERATIVE ACTION EXPERIMENTS **and their results.** Take note of what helped, what made things worse, and what produced no change. These details are gold for you and your practitioner to understand the underlying mechanisms of your symptoms. It's easy to forget the outcome of experiments over time, so write them down!

7

TREATING YOUR ROOT CAUSE

Once you've done Iterative Action Experiments on your foundations and run some testing to identify your deeper underlying root causes, it's time to do some Iterative Action treatment experiments to see if treatment improves your IBS symptoms.

This is an area where many IBS patients get quite lost in the weeds, and sadly, many practitioners may inadvertently mislead their patients as well. In this chapter, I want to share the high-level strategy tips that will help you get the most out of your gut infection treatments. You may need to advocate for yourself with your doctors if they're not totally up to date with these concepts.

Most of the treatments I will discuss in this chapter will require you to partner with a trusted doctor, specialist, naturopath, or other health practitioner, as many of them are prescriptions. For specific questions about prescription treatment, please reach out to your healthcare provider.

Order of Operations for Treating Infections

You may have found you have multiple underlying types of infections with your gut testing. What now? If this is your situation, first of all, don't panic! It's not that uncommon. It's also important to know how to best work on these causes in the right sequence.

Let's say you learned that you have SIBO, *H. pylori*, *Giardia* (a parasite), and Candida overgrowth (no wonder you have digestive symptoms!). In naturopathic medicine, these infections would be dealt with in this order: *H. pylori* first, *Giardia* (parasites) second, SIBO third, and Candida fourth. Why?

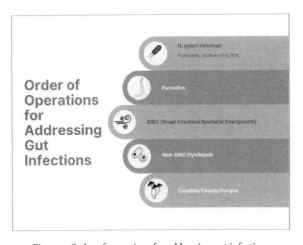

Figure 5: Order of operations for addressing gut infections.

Well, again, *H. pylori* infects the stomach. Because this is one of the most upstream parts of the digestive system, if it's not functioning well, *everything* downstream may be compromised. So if *H. pylori* and its symptoms are present, you'll want to address this first.

Then, if parasites are present, they come next. Parasites can really muck up the place, cause inflammation, and impede your treatment progress.

Next, bacteria. This includes SIBO, or non-SIBO dysbiosis, but not *H. pylori* (see above). Non-SIBO dysbiosis may not require specific medical treatment *per se*, but in any event, it comes next.

Finally, you tackle Candida or other yeast overgrowths. Often, addressing bacteria leaves Candida without any checks and balances. This is why it's common to have a yeast infection after a course of antibiotics.

However, it's important to keep in mind that even if you have all four types of infections, this *doesn't* mean you definitely need to address each one of them in turn directly. **Each round of treatment should be considered an Iterative Action Experiment, and part of that process is to evaluate how you're feeling once you complete the experiment.**

You may find that you feel well enough after the first round of treatment to stop direct treatment. This happened to my client Dave, whom I mentioned in Chapter 2. Once he treated his *H. pylori*, he felt well enough that he didn't need to treat the SIBO and other things that turned up on his testing.

It may seem odd not to treat what you found on paper. It's important to remember that a test result is just a number. You always want to correlate your results with your actual signs and symptoms. If you're SIBO positive but don't have any symptoms, you don't need to treat SIBO.

Ultimately, how you feel is your best guide to determine whether or not you need to pursue deeper treatment.

Treating *H. Pylori*

If it turns out that you have *H. pylori*, addressing this root cause may improve your entire digestive system.

Conventional *H. pylori* treatment is two weeks of "triple therapy," which includes two antibiotics (usually metronidazole, amoxicillin, or clarithromycin) and an over-the-counter proton pump inhibitor (PPI), such as Pepcid AC. Some doctors also include bismuth (Pepto-Bismol) as research suggests this may increase the protocol's effectiveness (Poonyam et. al., 2019).

There are several alternative methods for addressing *H. pylori*, but you should know there isn't much research to show they're effective. However, if the alternative treatment isn't harmful, it's reasonable to try an Iterative Action Experiment to see if it's effective for you. You can always try the conventional treatment in the future if the non-standard approach doesn't help.

Non-pharmaceutical options for *H. pylori* include:

- **Mastic gum and Berberine:** Mastic gum has been researched for its potential anti-bacterial effect on *H. pylori* specifically, but what initially looked like promising results were not repeated in larger-scale trials. However, mastic gum may still have some therapeutic effect on some cases of *H. pylori*. In supplements, it's often paired with berberine as a natural antibiotic. Usually, this is used for 30 days.
- **Matula tea:** Matula tea is a proprietary herb blend that is supposed to have a therapeutic effect on *H. pylori* infection. The tea is used twice a day for 30 days. The matula tea company offers a money-back guarantee if you can provide a post-treatment test showing a continued *H. pylori* infection after treatment.
- *Saccharomyces boulardii* **Probiotics:** There is some research to suggest that *Saccharomyces boulardii* probiotics can improve outcomes when used

alongside other *H. pylori* treatments, including antibiotics (Zhou et. al., 2019; Eslami et. al., 2019; Shi et. al., 2019). It may be helpful to include these probiotics no matter which treatment path you choose.

Just as with SIBO, it's important to retest after treatment to see whether your approach was successful or not. Depending on what you find, you'll create your next Iterative Action Experiment from there.

Treating Parasites

Parasites sometimes turn up as an underlying IBS cause for my clients. Most often, we see small, single-celled parasites, like amoebas, but worms are definitely a possibility too. However, testing positive for a parasite on your stool test doesn't necessarily mean that parasites are causing your problem.

As with anything you find on a lab test, you have to approach by asking the question, is this actually causing my symptoms? And the way you answer that question is by doing an Iterative Action treatment experiment to test your theory.

There are many different types of parasites, and their treatment will depend on you and the specific parasite. There are anti-parasite drugs you can use or herbal options as well. Drug treatment is typically very short-term (7 days or so), while herbal options are usually 30-60 days. You'll want to discuss this with your doctor.

Here are a few key tips for succeeding with parasite treatment.

- Because parasites have complex life cycles, it may be necessary to pulse treatment over several months to make sure you eradicate all the different life-cycle forms.

- A biofilm buster can often improve treatment outcomes, as parasites (and other microorganisms) can hide from treatment in biofilms.
- As with SIBO and *H. pylori*, retesting is important to confirm that you've successfully cleared your parasite infection. Make sure to use this follow-up test and your symptom improvement to help guide your next steps.

SIBO Treatment Tips

SIBO is one of the most likely infections for those with IBS symptoms. The good news is SIBO is a specifically treatable condition! However, succeeding with SIBO treatment requires some savvy strategy and specific steps.

Now let's talk about a strategy for SIBO treatment.

SIBO Treatment Strategy

There are five primary steps to addressing SIBO correctly:

1. Before treatment, reduce food triggers, reduce stress, and support your baseline gut function as much as possible.
2. Treat SIBO, either with antibiotics, antimicrobial herbs, or an elemental diet.
3. Follow-up treatment with a prokinetic agent (a medication or herbal formula that increases gut motility), starting as soon as you finish treatment.
4. Retest two weeks post-treatment.

5. Decide your next steps based on what you learned during and after your treatment.

Let's cover some important details about each step.

1. BEFORE TREATMENT, REDUCE FOOD TRIGGERS, STRESS, AND Support Gut Function:

If you haven't already done this before your SIBO diagnosis, identifying your food triggers can help you minimize your symptoms and teach you how to maintain that symptom relief. See Chapter 4 for a discussion about how to do this properly.

A note about your diet during SIBO treatment: Though many SIBO influencers recommend "eating normally while on SIBO treatment to feed the bacteria," I think minimizing your symptoms during treatment is important. If you're feeling better afterward, you can try food reintroductions to see if your tolerances have changed.

2. TREAT SIBO

There are three recognized ways of treating SIBO:

1. **Antibiotics:** A specialized antibiotic, Rifaximin (also known as Xifaxin) was developed to have action only in the small intestine and to minimize the negative side effects that we all associate with antibiotics. Rifaximin is used alone for hydrogen SIBO, in combination with Neomycin or Metronidazole for methane SIBO, and in combination with bismuth for hydrogen sulfide SIBO. Doctors typically prescribe the antibiotics for 14 days, but sometimes,

in stubborn cases, 21-30 days may be required at the discretion of your doctor.

2. **Herbal Antibiotics:** You can also treat SIBO with herbal antibiotics, including neem oil, berberine, oregano oil, and allicin, a garlic derivative. Research suggests that herbal SIBO treatments are as effective as pharmaceutical antibiotic treatment if used properly (Chedid et. al., 2014). Typically, a course is considered 30 days.

3. **Elemental Diet:** A third treatment option is the Elemental Diet, which uses a liquid, full-nutrition meal replacement containing no fiber. This starves the bacteria, treating the SIBO. According to research, 14 days of an elemental diet is as effective as antibiotics or herbal antimicrobials (Pimentel et. al., 2004).

It's important to know and expect that getting to full remission from SIBO may require multiple rounds of treatment. If you're starting with very high gas levels, you're more likely to need repeat courses of treatment. I personally needed *four courses* of antibiotic treatment to get my SIBO under control. Retesting after treatment is important to make sure that the overgrowth is managed and in full retreat. Be prepared to re-treat if necessary.

Additional supplements that may increase your success during SIBO treatment include:

- **Atrantil:** An herbal supplement that can help reduce methane-producing bacteria or archaea. See the Resources section.
- **Partially hydrolyzed guar gum (PHGG):** Also known as SunFiber, research suggests SIBO patients

who used this supplement during treatment had better treatment outcomes (Furnari et. al., 2010)

- **Biofilm buster:** Biofilm is a mucous coating that protects bacteria and other microorganisms from antimicrobial treatments. Biofilm busters are supplements that can eat away at this biofilm and may increase your treatment success. Examples of biofilm busters include N-Acetyl-Cysteine (NAC) and Biofilm Phase 2.

I expect SIBO treatment to evolve over the next few years, as at the time of this writing, Dr. Pimentel and his team are working on new and novel treatments for different types of SIBO.

3. FOLLOW-UP SIBO TREATMENT WITH PROKINETICS

The word *prokinetic* literally means "pro-movement," which tells you that this treatment improves the natural cleaning waves in your small intestine to keep the gut free from future SIBO flare-ups.

Prokinetic treatment should begin immediately after you finish your chosen SIBO treatment. Here are the most common options to discuss with your doctor, naturopath, or other medical provider:

- **Prucalopride (Motegrity)** is a serotonergic agonist, which are just fancy words to say it encourages the action of serotonin in your gut. Prucalopride very specifically enhances the natural cleaning waves in the small intestine and helps prevent SIBO relapse. It has also been prescribed for chronic constipation.

- **Low-Dose Erythromycin** is a low dose of an antibiotic that increases gut motility.
- **MotilPro from Pure Encapsulations** is a supplement that uses ginger, 5-HTP, and vitamin B6 as a prokinetic. However, some people do not tolerate dried ginger, so use it with caution.
- **Iberogast** is a liquid supplement that contains pro-motility herbs.
- **Motility Activator** by Integrative Therapeutics, and herbal supplement containing ginger and artichoke leaf extract.

There may be other options that your doctor or naturopath can offer you. For very stubborn cases, herbal options may not have enough therapeutic effect.

Prokinetics are typically taken at bedtime to enhance your strongest natural cleaning waves, which happen during your long overnight fast.

4. Retest Two Weeks After Treatment

Your SIBO treatment is essentially an Iterative Action Experiment asking, "Does SIBO treatment improve my digestive symptoms?" An important follow-up evaluation to this experiment is to run a repeat SIBO test. This retest is a unique opportunity to correlate your symptom changes with what happened to your actual gas levels.

What should you do with that retest data?

- If you saw symptom improvement and your gas levels decreased, this is a strong indicator that SIBO was causing your symptoms.

- If your symptoms didn't improve and your gas levels changed, this suggests that your symptoms are *not* related to SIBO and that you need to investigate other causes.
- If your symptoms improved and your gas levels changed but are still high, you're on the right track but you may need more treatment.

This is a crucial step, so if you're unsure what to do with your test results, connect with a knowledgeable practitioner.

5. DECIDE YOUR NEXT STEPS BASED ON WHAT YOU LEARNED

Using what you learned from your repeat test and your symptom changes, create your next round of Iterative Action Experiments. This may look like:

- Exploring how prokinetics affect you and dialing in the right dose.
- Creating a new Iterative Action Experiment to assess the role of another root cause (like Candida, for example).
- Treating for SIBO again, if indicated.
- Doing food reintroductions to explore whether your SIBO treatment changed your food intolerances.
- Testing digestive function supports, like probiotics, to see if they help.

As always, develop questions you need to answer, create new hypotheses about what's happening, and test things carefully, one at a time.

When you use this five-step SIBO strategy, you methodically experiment and grow your personal knowledge of what exactly will best help resolve your SIBO.

Treating Candida

If Candida turned up on your stool test, treatment is relatively simple but may require some dedication. Reducing sugar and alcohol consumption is a low-hanging fruit that is a very helpful foundation for addressing Candida, but sometimes more treatment is necessary.

Conventional antifungal treatment is typically done with antifungal drugs like Fluconazole or Nystatin, and often lasts 14-30 days. Herbal antifungal treatment agents include Uva ursi, caprylic acid, and grapefruit seed extract and are typically used for between 30 and 60 days.

Some interesting recent research suggests that pulsing antifungal treatment every two to three days may be more effective than continuous use. However, this research was done on toenail fungus infections, so may not apply to gut infections (Westerberg et. al., 2013).

As with other types of intestinal overgrowths and infections, biofilm busters may increase your success.

Fungal overgrowth can be a reason for increased symptoms during or after antibiotic treatment for infections like *H. pylori* and SIBO. If this happens to you, it can be worth discussing this possibility with your doctor to assess whether antifungal treatment might help take your healing to the next level.

Retesting for Candida with stool testing can help you assess whether your approach has been effective or not, and help you plan your next steps.

Treating Adhesions and Scar Tissue

If you have a health history that includes having been in accidents, abdominal surgeries, or endometriosis, one of your root causes may be adhesions and scar tissue. If this is the case, having long-term relief from your IBS demands you do what you can to address this.

It's difficult to confirm if you have adhesions or scar tissue short of having exploratory surgery. However, if your health history suggests they may be one of your root causes, hands-on therapy can be really helpful.

The option with the most results and research to back it up is the Clear Passage clinics, which are located throughout the US, as well as in the UK and Australia (See Resources for information on how to contact them). Specially trained physical therapists offer a unique intensive program of twenty hours of manual therapy in one week to massage, stretch, and break down scar tissue and adhesions in your abdominal cavity.

I completed the Clear Passage program of physical therapy in November of 2021 and have had some of the most meaningful progress yet with my IBS symptoms and food intolerances. As of this writing, almost a year later, I am still SIBO-free. After ten years of SIBO symptoms, I am so grateful for these results!

If you don't have access to or the budget for Clear Passage therapists, other options include finding physical therapists or craniosacral therapists who can safely do visceral therapy work to help.

The Power of Successfully Treating Root Causes

Treating infections or other root causes is often the last missing piece that finally relieves IBS patients' symptoms and suffering.

When my clients succeed with this step, we all feel so excited and happy. After months or years of struggle, they can finally breathe easily and imagine a different future for themselves.

Though there's no single roadmap for everyone that can accurately direct you on how to get here, using the Iterative Action Method to test the options and evaluate your individual response carefully is how you find relief.

When you finally arrive at the 'most root cause' and treatment that truly addresses what's most responsible for your symptoms, you'll feel so much better. When you find this for yourself, it's not only a relief to feel better, but it's also so exciting to feel like you figured out the puzzle.

So get curious, figure out which root cause makes the most sense, and test your theory.

8

MAINTAIN YOUR IBS SYMPTOM RELIEF

U p to this point, I've provided you with many possible experiments to try to help you get to the bottom of what's causing your IBS symptoms. So what do you need to do to maintain your IBS symptom relief?

In essence, you simply need to do what you've learned helps and continue avoiding what makes things worse. It really is that simple!

But as with all simple things, there are important details to remember. Though some of us get lucky with a one-and-done treatment, many of us (me included) may need to manage our symptoms with various tools in the long term to stay symptom-free.

So in this chapter, I'm going to share some tips and tricks for using the Iterative Action Method to maintain your symptom relief in the long term.

Over time, with the results and insights you've gained from your experiments, you begin to narrow down your options to a few solid things to work with that you know, *without a doubt,* improve your symptoms. Eventually, you're left with just a few things at the bottom of your funnel.

For each of you, the unique, specific steps you need to take to keep your bowels happy will be particular to you. To give you an example of what this looks like, here's what I've figured out through my many Iterative Action Experiments that I know helps me maintain my gut health.

1. I need to eat fiber at every meal to prevent constipation.
2. I need to avoid gluten, dairy, beef, and pork, no exceptions, to prevent abdominal pain, bloating, and diarrhea. There are other foods I need to eat only in moderation, like onions, garlic, spicy foods, and chard, to avoid bloating and back pain.
3. I supplement with quercetin, magnesium citrate, vitamin D, and amino acids. These encourage my gut motility and improve my histamine tolerance, as well as my mood.
4. I use prescription bioidentical hormone replacement. Now that I'm through menopause, it helps me maintain a balanced mood, sleep cycle, and healthy tissue tone. It also seems to improve my gut motility slightly.
5. Getting enough sleep and taking care of myself to reduce stress helps keep me healthy overall, including in my gut.

As long as I follow this program for myself, I'm functional again. I've worked it seamlessly into my daily routine, and it doesn't feel like extra work anymore. I can travel, and I understand my limitations. Best of all, I can pursue my passions and interests without being limited by my physical symptoms. Ultimately, this is what we do it for, right? You can do this, too.

Your Long-Term IBS Management Plan

Your long-term symptom management plan includes two things:

1. Do more of what clearly works and provides you with benefits.
2. Do less of what doesn't work or triggers symptoms.

It's as simple as that!

In addition, if you still aren't quite where you'd like to be, you can continue investigating any root causes using the Iterative Action Method.

You may never find a complete cure, but you can get close with a plan to maintain your symptom remission. It makes me think of this crazy concept in mathematics I remember from school. (Bear with me, this is a little nerdy!)

An *asymptote* is a curved graph from an equation that never reaches zero. As you progress along the curve, you get closer and closer to zero but will never actually arrive.

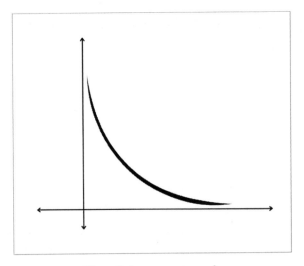

Figure X: An asymptote graph.

THIS IS OFTEN WHAT I FEEL IT'S LIKE IN IBS AND SIBO CASES. "Zero" would mean a complete cure.

In my personal case, I had SIBO and parasites that were causing digestive symptoms, but I also had endometriosis. As best as I can tell, the endometriosis and the adhesions it caused were the root cause of my slow motility that led to SIBO.

I kept thinking I had a thyroid problem, but repeated thyroid testing never showed a thyroid imbalance. I also had a severe case of amoebic dysentery when traveling in Nepal, which may have contributed. I'll never *really* know 100% exactly what caused my problem, but it doesn't really matter.

What I do know is enough to guide my treatment to maintain and prevent my symptoms, to get me as close to zero, or my complete cure, as possible.

Here are my top tips for maintaining your long-term IBS management plan.

. . .

Tip 1: Continue to avoid any trigger foods that continue
to cause symptoms! No one wants to avoid foods for the long
term, but if a food continues to cause problems, avoid it
without excuses.

What you can do here is continue to ask why you still have
this ongoing sensitivity and consider what you might do to
improve it. For example, I was unable to tolerate any bread at
all when my SIBO symptoms were at their worst. But when I
finally cleared SIBO, I could eat gluten-free bread without a
problem. It seems like the SIBO somehow affected my ability to
digest and break down those foods correctly. However, I still
can't eat more than a bite of dairy without serious consequences, so I don't eat it at all. Just use your body to guide you.

Tip 2: Continue any habit that improves your digestion,
and make it a permanent routine. Continuing the habits you
found made the biggest difference, like chewing slowly at every
meal, sipping less water while you're eating, relieving stress
with meditations or hypnosis, moving your body, or supporting
your digestive functions with supplements.

Tip 3: Periodically reconfirm you need to continue your
actions. Some methods, techniques, food eliminations, supplements, or medications don't need to be used forever. You can
complete Iterative Action Experiments by *removing* something
to see if you still feel well without it. For example, you can try
stopping probiotics to see if your symptoms stay on track
without them. If so, then you've just saved yourself some
money. If not, then you can continue using them. You only need
to continue to do practices that *actually show benefit* for
your gut.

. . .

TIP 4: IF YOUR SYMPTOMS RETURN, FALL BACK ON WHAT YOU learned from your Iterative Action Experiments. Revisit the Iterative Action Method, ask new questions about the likely underlying mechanisms of your symptoms, and use the process to discover new possibilities to help you.

TIP 5: WRITE DOWN YOUR MAINTENANCE PLAN TO HELP YOU STAY on track. When you get clear about what helps you, note it on a list, and post it in a visible place, like your refrigerator. This way, you can keep your discoveries in the front of your mind.

Your Life After Digestive Symptoms

I know your efforts can feel futile, like you'll never arrive. I also know it wouldn't be unusual for you to feel frustrated with your slow progress or overwhelmed with all the options. And in some of those moments, you might be tempted to throw your hands up and throw in the towel.

If you're feeling like this, I can totally empathize. I certainly had dark moments during my process where I was worried that whatever was causing my symptoms might kill me and leave my kids motherless. And many of my clients walk through my door feeling the same.

But what I want to leave you with is a sense that there *are* paths forward by relying on process and creative thinking. You *can* find the solutions that will help you re-emerge from your cloistered IBS life.

There *is* a life ahead for you where you can book a trip without anxiety about what will happen with your gut on the plane or at the hotel. A life where you can go out to eat and trust that you'll be fine afterward. A life where you have the energy to play with your kids or grandkids or go out on a date with your partner. A life where you don't feel anxious every time you look inside the refrigerator.

Even better, there is a life ahead where you can follow your passions, do well in your chosen career, or delight in feeling well.

It may not happen overnight, and getting there may not be easy. But it *is* possible. Imagine what opportunities would be available if your digestion no longer ruled your life.

If you're willing to apply the strategy and process I shared in this book, I believe this is possible for you .

It can take a moment to realize you've succeeded. Last year, a few months after my successful SIBO treatment process, I decided to make chocolate chip cookies. I couldn't tolerate gluten-free flour, eggs, or chocolate when I was sick.

Because of this, I hadn't eaten a chocolate chip cookie in about five years. This cost me dearly. Not only do I love cookies, but I stopped baking with my kids. It was just sad for me to help them with the process but not be able to enjoy the cookies at the end.

But one day last spring, I made a batch of cookies and savored not only baking them, but sinking my teeth into them and crunching up those chocolate chips. It felt like this one moment opened up the whole world again. I had options and possibilities I had missed for a long time. You can have this moment, too.

It may require you to try new things, change your diet, or try new supplements or treatments. You may have moments of uncertainty. But I promise you that if you apply this method of action and experimentation, creative thinking, and of trying to understand the why underneath everything that happens, you will eventually find the useful answers you crave.

Whatever you find, it will be perfectly unique to you, created by your own inquiry and results.

So start creating your unique and custom calm digestion plan by applying the Iterative Action Method. Get curious, and find what your precious digestive system needs to feel well, so that you can get back to life in full. There *is* life after digestive symptoms, and you can live it. What will you do with your life when your gut is happy again?

RESOURCES

Here are select resources to help you find things I discussed in the book. Please note that some of these links are affiliate links, meaning that if you purchase the product, I will receive a small commission at no additional cost to you. Thank you for supporting my small, woman-owned business!

IBS and SIBO Coaching Support with Amanda:

- I currently support clients in an online coaching program called The Calm Digestion Method. To inquire about working together, please visit https://helpforibsandsibo.com.

IBS Testing

- IBSSmart test: https://ibssmart.com

SIBO Testing

- Trio-Smart Test: https://triosmartbreath.com
- Life Extension: https://www.lifeextension.com/lab-testing/itemlc100063/sibo-home-breath-kit-lactulose
- FoodMarble AIRE 2: https://foodmarble.com/shop

Stool Testing

- **Diagnostic Solutions Laboratory (GI MAP):** https://diagnosticsolutionslab.com. Call their toll-free customer service number to request clinician referrals in your area.
- **Parasites.org Precise Home Parasite Test:**https://www.parasites.org/home-stool-test-kit-for-human-parasites-confluence-nutrition/

Nervous System Retraining:

- Dynamic Neural Retraining System (DNRS): https://www.dnrsonline.com/
- The Gupta Program: https://www.guptaprogram.com/aff/264/
- Eye Movement and Desensitization and Reprocessing (EMDR) Therapy: https://www.emdria.org/find-an-emdr-therapist/
- Emotional Freedom Technique (EFT): https://eftinternational.org/wp-content/uploads/EFT-International-Free-Tapping-Manual.pdf

Elemental Heal from Dr. Ruscio's Functional Medicine Formulations:

- **Regular Formula:** https://store.drruscio.com/products/elemental-heal
- **Whey-free Formula:** https://store.drruscio.com/products/elemental-heal-whey-free
- **Low-Carb Formula:** https://store.drruscio.com/products/elemental-heal-low-carb
- **Elemental Heal Dosing Calculator:** https://drruscio.com/eh-dosing-calculator/

Mold Referrals:

- Navigating Mold Toxicity and Treatment: https://drruscio.com/navigating-mold-toxicity-treatment/
- Simple But Effective Treatment of Mold Toxicity: https://drruscio.com/treatment-of-mold-toxicity/

Atrantil: https://atrantil.com

Clear Passage Therapy:
https://clearpassage.com

BIBLIOGRAPHY

Besirbellioglu, B. A., Ulcay, A., Can, M., Erdem, H., Tanyuksel, M., Avci, I. Y., Araz, E., & Pahsa, A. (2006). Saccharomyces boulardii and infection due to Giardia lamblia. *Scandinavian journal of infectious diseases*, *38*(6-7), 479–481. https://doi.org/10.1080/00365540600561769

Blood test for IBS. (n.d.). Blood test for IBS | Diagnose IBS. Ibs-Smart. Retrieved September 13, 2022, from https://www.ibssmart.com/

Bolen, B. (2022, July 19). Learn if a candida overgrowth is causing your IBS. Verywell Health. https://www.verywellhealth.com/ibs-and-candida-1944737

Breit, S., Kupferberg, A., Rogler, G., & Hasler, G. (2018). Vagus nerve as a modulator of the brain-gut axis in psychiatric and inflammatory disorders. Frontiers in Psychiatry, 9(44). https://doi.org/10.3389/fpsyt.2018.00044

Brennan, D. D. (2021, July 1). What to know about prokinetic agents. WebMD. https://www.webmd.com/heartburn-gerd/what-to-know-prokinetic-agents

Carek, P. J., Laibstain, S. E., & Carek, S. M. (2011). Exercise for the treatment of depression and anxiety. The International Journal of Psychiatry in Medicine, 41(1), 15–28. https://doi.org/10.2190/pm.41.1.c

Chiaffarino, F., Cipriani, S., Ricci, E., Mauri, P. A., Esposito, G., Barretta, M., Vercellini, P., & Parazzini, F. (2021). Endometriosis and irritable bowel syndrome: a systematic review and meta-analysis. *Archives of gynecology and obstetrics*, *303*(1), 17–25. https://doi.org/10.1007/s00404-020-05797-8

Chedid, V., Dhalla, S., Clarke, J. O., Roland, B. C., Dunbar, K. B., Koh, J., Justino, E., Tomakin, E., & Mullin, G. E. (2014). Herbal therapy is equivalent to rifaximin for the treatment of small intestinal bacterial overgrowth. *Global advances in health and medicine*, *3*(3), 16–24. https://doi.org/10.7453/gahmj.2014.019

Cho-Dorado, M. (2017, December 19). Steatorrhea: causes, symptoms, and treatment. Www.medicalnewstoday.com. https://www.medicalnewstoday.com/articles/320361

Cox, S. R., Lindsay, J. O., Fromentin, S., Stagg, A. J., McCarthy, N. E., Galleron, N., Ibraim, S. B., Roume, H., Levenez, F., Pons, N., Maziers, N., Lomer, M. C., Ehrlich, S. D., Irving, P. M., & Whelan, K. (2020). Effects of Low FODMAP Diet on Symptoms, Fecal Microbiome, and Markers of Inflammation in Patients With Quiescent Inflammatory Bowel Disease in a

Randomized Trial. *Gastroenterology*, *158*(1), 176–188.e7. https://doi.org/10. 1053/j.gastro.2019.09.024

Denhard, Dr. M. (2022, February 10). Digestive enzymes and digestive enzyme supplements. Www.hopkinsmedicine.org. https://www.hopkinsmedicine. org/health/wellness-and-prevention/digestive-enzymes-and-digestive-enzyme-supplements#:~:text=You

Dube, S. R., Fairweather, D., Pearson, W. S., Felitti, V. J., Anda, R. F., & Croft, J. B. (2009). Cumulative childhood stress and autoimmune diseases in adults. *Psychosomatic medicine*, *71*(2), 243–250. https://doi.org/10.1097/PSY. 0b013e3181907888

Endometriosis. (n.d.). Endometriosis. John Hopkins Medicine. Retrieved September 20, 2022, from https://www.hopkinsmedicine.org/health/condi tions-and-diseases/endometrios,is#:~:text=Endometriosis%20Definition

Eslami, M., Yousefi, B., Kokhaei, P., Jazayeri Moghadas, A., Sadighi Moghadam, B., Arabkari, V., & Niazi, Z. (2019). Are probiotics useful for therapy of Helicobacter pylori diseases?. *Comparative immunology, microbiology and infectious diseases*, *64*, 99–108. https://doi.org/10.1016/j.cimid.2019. 02.010

Fast tract diet for SIBO and IBS. (n.d.). The fast tract diet for SIBO and IBS. Meredith East Powell Brisbane Nutrition, Yoga and Mentoring. Retrieved September 14, 2022, from https://www.mereditheastpowell.com/blog/the-fast-tract-diet-for-sibo-and-ibs

Ford, A. C., Quigley, E. M., Lacy, B. E., Lembo, A. J., Saito, Y. A., Schiller, L. R., Soffer, E. E., Spiegel, B. M., & Moayyedi, P. (2014). Efficacy of prebiotics, probiotics, and synbiotics in irritable bowel syndrome and chronic idio-pathic constipation: systematic review and meta-analysis. *The American journal of gastroenterology*, *109*(10), 1547–1562. https://doi.org/10.1038/ajg. 2014.202

Furnari, M., Parodi, A., Gemignani, L., Giannini, E. G., Marenco, S., Savarino, E., Assandri, L., Fazio, V., Bonfanti, D., Inferrera, S., & Savarino, V. (2010). Clinical trial: the combination of rifaximin with partially hydrolysed guar gum is more effective than rifaximin alone in eradicating small intestinal bacterial overgrowth. *Alimentary pharmacology & therapeutics*, *32*(8), 1000–1006. https://doi.org/10.1111/j.1365-2036.2010.04436.x

Ghoshal, U. C., Shukla, R., & Ghoshal, U. (2017). Small intestinal bacterial overgrowth and irritable bowel syndrome: A bridge between functional organic dichotomy. Gut and Liver, 11(2), 196–208.

Gibson, P. R., & Shepherd, S. J. (2010). Evidence-based dietary management of functional gastrointestinal symptoms: The FODMAP approach. *Journal of gastroenterology and hepatology*, 25(2), 252–258. https://doi.org/10.1111/j.1440-1746.2009.06149.x

Gibson P. R. (2017). Use of the low-FODMAP diet in inflammatory bowel disease. *Journal of gastroenterology and hepatology*, *32 Suppl 1*, 40–42. https://doi.org/10.1111/jgh.13695

GI-MAP. (2022, August 21). GI-MAP. GI Microbial Assay Plus. Diagnostic Solutions Laboratory. https://www.diagnosticsolutionslab.com/tests/gi-map

Gut health quotes. (n.d.). Gut health quotes (20 quotes). Www.goodreads.com. https://www.goodreads.com/quotes/tag/gut-health

Gut-brain connection. (2021, April 19). The gut-brain connection. Harvard Health. https://www.health.harvard.edu/diseases-and-conditions/the-gut-brain-connection#:~:text=A%20troubled%20intestine%20can%20send

Halpin, S. J., & Ford, A. C. (2012). Prevalence of symptoms meeting criteria for Irritable Bowel Syndrome in Inflammatory Bowel Disease: Systematic Review and Meta-Analysis. American Journal of Gastroenterology, 107(10), 1474–1482. https://doi.org/10.1038/ajg.2012.260

Hedin, C., Whelan, K., & Lindsay, J. O. (2007). Evidence for the use of probiotics and prebiotics in inflammatory bowel disease: a review of clinical trials. *The Proceedings of the Nutrition Society*, 66(3), 307–315. https://doi.org/10.1017/S0029665107005563

https://pubmed.ncbi.nlm.nih.gov/22929759/

IBS facts and statistics. (2007). IBS facts and statistics. International Foundation for Gastrointestinal Disorders. https://aboutibs.org/what-is-ibs/facts-about-ibs/

IBS vs IBD. (2020, April 1). IBS vs IBD. Beth Israel Deaconess Medical Centre. https://www.bidmc.org/about-bidmc/wellness-insights/gastrointestinal-gi-health/2016/04/ibs-vs-ibd#:~:text=IBS%20is%20a%20chronic%20syndrome

Jerkunica, E. (n.d.). Parasites that cause IBS symptoms. Parasites.org. Retrieved September 20, 2022, from https://www.parasites.org/ibs-symptoms/

Kim, B., Park, Y., Kim, B., Ahn, H. J., Lee, K. A., Chung, J. E., & Han, S. W. (2019). Diagnostic performance of CA 125, HE4, and risk of Ovarian Malignancy Algorithm for ovarian cancer. *Journal of clinical laboratory analysis*, 33(1), e22624. https://doi.org/10.1002/jcla.22624

Kruis, W., Fric, P., Pokrotnieks, J., Lukás, M., Fixa, B., Kascák, M., Kamm, M. A., Weismueller, J., Beglinger, C., Stolte, M., Wolff, C., & Schulze, J. (2004). Maintaining remission of ulcerative colitis with the probiotic Escherichia coli Nissle 1917 is as effective as with standard mesalazine. *Gut, 53*(11), 1617–1623. https://doi.org/10.1136/gut.2003.037747

Kvarnstrom, H. (2018, June 21). Exploring common conditions misdiagnosed as IBS and why diagnostic accuracy is essential. Alternative Medicine Review. https://altmedrev.com/blog/exploring-common-conditions-misdi agnosed-as-ibs-and-why-diagnostic-accuracy-is-essential/

Larson, J. (2022, June 22). This is what stomach pain could be telling you about type 1 diabetes. Healthline. https://www.healthline.com/health/ diabetes/type-1-diabetes-stomach-pain#gastroparesis

Leeds, J. S., Hopper, A. D., Sidhu, R., Simmonette, A., Azadbakht, N., Hoggard, N., Morley, S., & Sanders, D. S. (2010). Some patients with irritable bowel syndrome may have exocrine pancreatic insufficiency. Clinical Gastroenterology and Hepatology, 8(5), 433–438. https://doi.org/10.1016/j.cgh.2009. 09.032

Li, Chenyu BSa,c; Shuai, Yujun BSa,c; Zhou, Xiaodong PhDa; Chen, Hongxia PhDb. Association between Helicobacter pylori infection and irritable bowel syndrome: A systematic review and meta-analysis. Medicine: December 11, 2020 - Volume 99 - Issue 50 - p e2297. 5doi: 10.1097/MD.0000000000022975

Liew, W. P., & Mohd-Redzwan, S. (2018). Mycotoxin: Its Impact on Gut Health and Microbiota. *Frontiers in cellular and infection microbiology, 8*, 60. https:// doi.org/10.3389/fcimb.2018.00060

McMahon, L. (2022, January 12). The low fermentation diet for SIBO. Epicured. https://blog.epicured.com/low-fermentation-sibo

Muizzuddin, N., Maher, W., Sullivan, M., Schnittger, S., & Mammone, T. (2012). Physiological effect of a probiotic on skin. *Journal of cosmetic science, 63*(6), 385–395.

Ng, Q. X., Peters, C., Ho, C., Lim, D. Y., & Yeo, W. S. (2018). A meta-analysis of the use of probiotics to alleviate depressive symptoms. *Journal of affective disorders, 228*, 13–19. https://doi.org/10.1016/j.jad.2017.11.063

Ogobuiro, I., Gonzales, J., & Tuma, F. (2022, April 21). Physiology, Gastrointestinal. PubMed; StatPearls Publishing.

Pedersen, N., Ankersen, D. V., Felding, M., Wachmann, H., Végh, Z., Molzen, L., Burisch, J., Andersen, J. R., & Munkholm, P. (2017). Low-FODMAP diet reduces irritable bowel symptoms in patients with inflammatory bowel disease. *World journal of gastroenterology, 23*(18), 3356–3366. https://doi.org/ 10.3748/wjg.v23.i18.3356

Pimentel, M., Soffer, E. E., Chow, E. J., Kong, Y., & Lin, H. C. (2002). Lower frequency of MMC is found in IBS subjects with abnormal lactulose breath test, suggesting bacterial overgrowth. *Digestive diseases and sciences*, 47(12), 2639–2643. https://doi.org/10.1023/a:1021039032413

Pimentel, M., Constantino, T., Kong, Y., Bajwa, M., Rezaei, A., & Park, S. (2004). A 14-day elemental diet is highly effective in normalizing the lactulose breath test. *Digestive diseases and sciences*, 49(1), 73–77. https://doi.org/10.1023/b:ddas.0000011605.43979.e1

Poonyam, P., Chotivitayatarakorn, P., & Vilaichone, R. K. (2019). High Effective of 14-Day High-Dose PPI- Bismuth-Containing Quadruple Therapy with Probiotics Supplement for Helicobacter Pylori Eradication: A Double Blinded-Randomized Placebo-Controlled Study. *Asian Pacific journal of cancer prevention : APJCP*, 20(9), 2859–2864. https://doi.org/10.31557/APJCP.2019.20.9.2859

Rome Foundation. (2016, January 16). C. Bowel disorders. Rome Foundation. https://theromefoundation.org/rome-iv/rome-iv-criteria/

Ruscio, Dr. M. (2020b, October 9). What are probiotics? Your guide to healthy gut bacteria. Drruscio.com. https://drruscio.com/what-are-probiotics/

Ruscio, Dr. M. (2021a, March 12). Mold toxicity, mold illness, and chronic symptoms. Dr. Ruscio. https://drruscio.com/mold-toxicity/

Sainsbury, A., Sanders, D. S., & Ford, A. C. (2013). Prevalence of irritable bowel syndrome-type symptoms in patients with celiac disease: a meta-analysis. Clinical Gastroenterology and Hepatology: The Official Clinical Practice Journal of the American Gastroenterological Association, 11(4), 359-365.e1. https://doi.org/10.1016/j.cgh.2012.11.033

Sarna, S. (2021). Healing SIBO: fix the real cause of IBS, bloating, and weight issues in 21 days (pp. 1–11). Avery, An Imprint Of Penguin Random House.

Seladi-Schulman, J. (2022, July 22). Vagus nerve: anatomy and function, diagram, stimulation, conditions. Healthline. https://www.healthline.com/human-body-maps/vagus-nerve

Sherwood, A. (2022, August 8). Specific Carbohydrate Diet (SCD diet): reviewing how it works. WebMD. https://www.webmd.com/ibd-crohns-disease/crohns-disease/specific-carbohydrate-diet-overview

Shi, X., Zhang, J., Mo, L., Shi, J., Qin, M., & Huang, X. (2019). Efficacy and safety of probiotics in eradicating Helicobacter pylori: A network meta-analysis. *Medicine*, 98(15), e15180. https://doi.org/10.1097/MD.0000000000015180

Siebecker, Dr. A. (n.d.). SIBO - Small Intestine Bacterial Overgrowth. SIBO - Small Intestine Bacterial Overgrowth. https://www.siboinfo.com/

Sonu, S., Post, S., & Feinglass, J. (2019). Adverse childhood experiences and the onset of chronic disease in young adulthood. Preventive Medicine, 123(30904602), 163–170. https://doi.org/10.1016/j.ypmed.2019.03.032

Staller, K., Olén, O., Söderling, J., Roelstraete, B., Törnblom, H., Khalili, H., Song, M., & Ludvigsson, J. F. (2021). Diagnostic yield of endoscopy in irritable bowel syndrome: A nationwide prevalence study 1987-2016. *European journal of internal medicine*, *94*, 85–92. https://doi.org/10.1016/j.ejim.2021.08.001

Steinbock, D. (2021, May 29). The gut-brain connection: how stress affects digestion. Mindful Family Medicine. https://mindfulfamilymedicine.com/the-gut-brain-connection-how-stress-affects-digestion/

Takakura, W., & Pimentel, M. (2020). Small Intestinal Bacterial Overgrowth and Irritable Bowel Syndrome – An Update. Frontiers in Psychiatry, 11(32754068). PubMed Central. https://doi.org/10.3389/fpsyt.2020.00664

Thorpe, M. (2017, March 8). 10 signs and symptoms of hypothyroidism. Healthline. https://www.healthline.com/nutrition/hypothyroidism-symptoms#constipation

Tiequn, B., Guanqun, C., & Shuo, Z. (2015). Therapeutic effects of Lactobacillus in treating irritable bowel syndrome: a meta-analysis. *Internal medicine (Tokyo, Japan)*, *54*(3), 243–249. https://doi.org/10.2169/internalmedicine.54.2710

Upper endoscopy. (2019, January 14). Upper endoscopy | EGD. American Cancer Society. https://www.cancer.org/treatment/understanding-your-diagnosis/tests/endoscopy/upper-endoscopy.html#:~:text=You%20are%20having%20problems%20in

van der Kolk, B. (2015). The Body Keeps the Score: Mind, Brain and Body in the Transformation of Trauma (p. 2). Penguin Books.

Veloso, H. G. (n.d.). FODMAP diet: what you need to know. Www.hopkinsmedicine.org. https://www.hopkinsmedicine.org/health/wellness-and-prevention/fodmap-diet-what-you-need-to-know

Wang, Z., He, Y., & Zheng, Y. (2019). Probiotics for the Treatment of Bacterial Vaginosis: A Meta-Analysis. *International journal of environmental research and public health*, *16*(20), 3859. https://doi.org/10.3390/ijerph16203859

Weitsman, S., Celly, S., Leite, G., Mathur, R., Sedighi, R., Barlow, G. M., Morales, W., Sanchez, M., Parodi, G., Villanueva-Millan, M. J., Rezaie, A., & Pimentel, M. (2022). Effects of Proton Pump Inhibitors on the Small Bowel and Stool Microbiomes. *Digestive diseases and sciences*, *67*(1), 224–232. https://doi.org/10.1007/s10620-021-06857-y

Westerberg, D. P., & Voyack, M. J. (2013). Onychomycosis: Current trends in diagnosis and treatment. *American family physician*, *88*(11), 762–770.

Whelan K. (2011). Probiotics and prebiotics in the management of irritable bowel syndrome: a review of recent clinical trials and systematic reviews. *Current opinion in clinical nutrition and metabolic care, 14*(6), 581–587. https://doi.org/10.1097/MCO.0b013e32834b8082

Yuan, F., Ni, H., Asche, C. V., Kim, M., Walayat, S., & Ren, J. (2017). Efficacy of Bifidobacterium infantis 35624 in patients with irritable bowel syndrome: a meta-analysis. *Current medical research and opinion, 33*(7), 1191–1197. https://doi.org/10.1080/03007995.2017.1292230

Zahedi, M. J., Behrouz, V., & Azimi, M. (2018). Low fermentable oligo-di-mono-saccharides and polyols diet versus general dietary advice in patients with diarrhea-predominant irritable bowel syndrome: A randomized controlled trial. *Journal of gastroenterology and hepatology, 33*(6), 1192–1199. https://doi.org/10.1111/jgh.14051

Zhan, Y. L., Zhan, Y. A., & Dai, S. X. (2018). Is a low FODMAP diet beneficial for patients with inflammatory bowel disease? A meta-analysis and systematic review. *Clinical nutrition (Edinburgh, Scotland), 37*(1), 123–129. https://doi.org/10.1016/j.clnu.2017.05.019

Zhang, C., Jiang, J., Tian, F., Zhao, J., Zhang, H., Zhai, Q., & Chen, W. (2020). Meta-analysis of randomized controlled trials of the effects of probiotics on functional constipation in adults. *Clinical nutrition (Edinburgh, Scotland), 39*(10), 2960–2969. https://doi.org/10.1016/j.clnu.2020.01.005

Zhong, C., Qu, C., Wang, B., Liang, S., & Zeng, B. (2017). Probiotics for Preventing and Treating Small Intestinal Bacterial Overgrowth: A Meta-Analysis and Systematic Review of Current Evidence. *Journal of clinical gastroenterology, 51*(4), 300–311. https://doi.org/10.1097/MCG.0000000000000814

Zhou, B. G., Chen, L. X., Li, B., Wan, L. Y., & Ai, Y. W. (2019). Saccharomyces boulardii as an adjuvant therapy for Helicobacter pylori eradication: A systematic review and meta-analysis with trial sequential analysis. *Helicobacter, 24*(5), e12651. https://doi.org/10.1111/hel.12651

ACKNOWLEDGMENTS

I've dreamed all my life of writing a book, and now I've gone and done it! But I certainly couldn't have done it alone.

Thank you so much for reading. If you enjoyed this book, I invite you to please leave a review on Amazon, as it truly does help more people find the book.

I'd like to thank many of the people who have contributed to my development, writing, and the production of this book.

First and foremost, I want to thank and acknowledge my husband Drew, and my dear kids, for being patient with me while I have dedicated a lot of my time to helping others, writing this book, and developing my health coaching business. I could not have accomplished everything I have without you.

I'd like to thank my wider family for encouraging all my hare-brained ideas.

A huge thank you to all my clients, and the people I have interviewed over the years, for sharing your stories so that I could learn what I needed to do to help others in your shoes.

A giant thank you to the practitioners, coaches, and teachers I have looked up to, and who have taught me what I need to know to be a helpful guide for others: Andrea Nakayama, Reed Davis, Joshua Rosenthal, Dr. Michael Ruscio,

Dr. Mark Pimentel, Dr. Ali Rezaie, Dr. Alison Siebecker, and countless others who have inspired me.

I'd like to thank my second families, Karl, Vanessa, Kai, and Kira, and Jeff, Susan, Larkyn, and Jasper, for always believing in me and rooting me on, and sharing your energetic support from afar.

I'd like to thank the Yang family, especially Hal and Georgia, for introducing me to the concept of coaching, and for being a stand for my potential, even when I couldn't see it myself.

I'd like to thank Kate Yang, my intrepid best friend, nine years gone now, who always encouraged me to reach for my dreams, even if it seemed ridiculous or impossible. Every time I do something big, I feel you with me.

Thank you to Caroline Wagenaar for always improving my writing, and editing this manuscript.

Thank you to The Urban Writers for providing copy editing for this book.

I want to thank the Audiobook Impact Academy and the Mikkelsen twins for teaching me how to write and publish a book, and for giving me the final push over the line to complete this dream.

And most of all, I want to thank you, dear reader, for taking a chance on reading what I have to say. May you find the missing clues and support you need to finally beat your IBS.

ABOUT THE AUTHOR

Amanda Malachesky is a former IBS sufferer who became determined to reframe the conventional approach to IBS after her own doctors failed her. Amanda is a Certified Functional Nutrition Health Coach, and has a Master's Degree in Ecological Design. She's the host of The Calm Digestion Method online coaching program that helps IBS and SIBO patients find their personalized IBS relief plan that works, and the Confluence Nutrition YouTube channel. She lives on California's Lost Coast with her family.

facebook.com/confluencenutrition

instagram.com/confluencenutrition26

youtube.com/confluencenutrition

Printed in Great Britain
by Amazon

30410175R00088